ISO 14001 Environmental Certification Step by Step

ISO 14001 Environmental Certification Step by Step

Revised first edition

A.J. Edwards

ELSEVIER
BUTTERWORTH
HEINEMANN

AMSTERDAM BOSTON HEIDELBERG LONDON NEW YORK OXFORD
PARIS SAN DIEGO SAN FRANCISCO SINGAPORE SYDNEY TOKYO

Elsevier Butterworth-Heinemann
Linacre House, Jordan Hill, Oxford OX2 8DP
200 Wheeler Road, Burlington MA 01803

First published 2001
Revised first edition 2004

British Library Cataloguing in Publication Data
A catalogue record for this book is available from the British Library

Library of Congress Cataloging in Publication Data
A catalogue record for this book is available from the Library of Congress

ISBN 0 7506 6100 3

For information on all Elsevier Butterworth-Heinemann publications
visit our website at: www.bh.com

Composition by Genesis Typesetting Limited, Rochester, Kent
Printed and bound in Italy

Contents

Preface to the revised edition

ISO 14001 Environmental Certification Step by Step was first published in April 2001, and was based on the information available and the understanding of the ISO 14001 Standard as in the latter part of 2000.

Now, two and a half years further on, there have been continuing developments in the following areas:

- international concern for the environment;
- new environmental legislation and changes to existing legislation;
- a greater understanding of how the Standard is being interpreted by the assessing bodies;
- changes to supporting information, e.g. sources of assistance;
- new supporting Standards.

The main international event was the World Summit on Sustainable Development in Johannesburg in 2002, a follow-up to the Rio World Summit of 1992.

New legislation is always coming on to the Statute Book. For example, the implementation of the *Pollution Prevention and Control Act 1999* is well advanced, replacing the *Environmental Protection Act 1990: Part 1*. New recycling initiatives are in the pipeline, such as the European Directives on end-of-life vehicles, tyres, electrical and electronic equipment, and batteries. The *Control of Pollution (Oil Storage) Regulations* make good practice mandatory.

Regarding the ISO 14001 Standard, experience shows that greater attention should be paid to:

- the setting of environmental objectives and targets and making progress towards their achievement;
- storage and the risks of pollution through poor handling practices or leakage;
- the control of contractors. It is surprising how many environmental incidents are caused by contractors working on someone else's premises;
- the procedures for communicating with employees, suppliers and contractors, the regulators and the public;
- training, particularly what to do when there is an emergency.

The opportunity has been taken to update the appendices, including new legislation, more sources of information and a significant increase in the number of assessing bodies accredited to assess to ISO 14001.

Preface to the revised edition

The results of a survey carried out for the Environment Agency and published at the end of 2002 revealed a general lack of environmental awareness among the UK's small and medium sized enterprises (SMEs). It was discouraging to find that 86% of the businesses interviewed did not think that their activities could harm the environment in any way, and that only 18% could name the environmental legislation that applied to them.

Even if your organisation decides it does not want to go all the way to registration to ISO 14001, it is my hope that this book will help you define your environmental responsibilities and impacts and give guidance on how you can keep control of them.

Tony Edwards
Lisvane, Cardiff

Preface

Concern for the environment is growing day by day. Damage to the environment is caused by our ever increasing demands which consume the world's natural resources, and by the pollution of land, water and air caused by our activities and the wastes we create.

More and more companies are seeking to understand how their operations impact on the environment, and these companies then put management systems in place to keep control of the impacts. Their concern is extending from their own activities to those of their suppliers and subcontractors; 'green' companies want to trade with 'green' partners.

An organisation's commitment to the environment and good environmental practice can now be demonstrated by being registered to ISO 14001, the international standard for environmental management systems. Organisations already registered to ISO 9001 will have no difficulty in recognising the model, but ISO 14001 has two important additional features: organisations must identify the environmental aspects inherent in their activities and define the impacts they have on the environment, and they must identify and obey any environmental legislation which applies to them. Then, following the ISO 9001 model, operating procedures need to be written and implemented together with a manual describing the environmental management system, before an independent assessment of compliance with the standard can take place.

This book is written primarily for small and medium sized enterprises who have decided that they want to create their own environmental management system as simply as possible whilst still being comprehensive.

Taking that good intention as the starting point, the book sets out the overall programme and then guides the reader through each step up to the time when the assessor leaves, hopefully with the words 'I am recommending you for registration to ISO 14001'.

The book includes model Registers of Environmental Aspects and Environmental Legislation, a model Environmental Management Manual and model Operating Procedures. Whilst the book is written so that it can be used by anyone who has no prior knowledge of documented management systems, where the requirements of the standard are similar to those of ISO 9001 the reader is encouraged to integrate the two systems into one.

As the range of possible environmental aspects and legislation is wide, it would not have been feasible to address every possibility. The book and its supplements include the most common aspects and regulations and examples of many others. There should be sufficient material for every reader to find either an actual text or a model which can be adapted to suit their own circumstances. Take heart from the fact that the number of organisations that have difficult environmental processes is quite small. For most people, control of waste arisings and its disposal, minimising energy and water consumption, good housekeeping and maybe packaging are likely to be the most significant aspects.

Preface

This book is accompanied by a website which includes downloadable versions of the model texts, Registers, Operating Procedures and Environmental Management Manual. The website is freely accessible to all purchasers of the book following a simple registration procedure. To access the files please visit www.books.elsevier.com/companions/0750661003 and follow the instructions on screen. The model texts are designed to make the process of copying and adaptation easier.

The model texts are all based on proven real life examples. I wish you the reader every success.

Tony Edwards
Lisvane, Cardiff

Acknowledgements

I gratefully acknowledge the input to this book provided by my colleagues in Penarth Management and the hard work of Mrs Judi Starling and Mrs Margaret Day in typing the script.

I also acknowledge the willingness of Alcatel Telecom Limited, Bartondale Engineering Company Limited, Geo Kingsbury MHP Machine Tools Limited, J Reid Trading Limited, Sonoco Industrial Products and Warwick International Limited to allow me to use material derived from their activities when writing the registers and operating procedures which support the book.

Lastly, but by no means the least, my thanks are due to Mr Fred Dobb, Commercial Manager, United Registrar of Systems, the author of the first volume in the series, who willingly allowed me to draw on relevant material from his book and then kindly reviewed the final text and made helpful suggestions for its improvement.

Extracts from the British Standard BS EN ISO 14001: 1996 are reproduced with the permission of BSI under licence number 2000SK/0399. Complete British Standards can be obtained by post from BSI Customer Services, 389 Chiswick High Road, London W4 4AL, UK, tel. +44 (0)20 8996 9001.

About the author

The author has had a long career in heavy industry followed by nearly ten years working as a consultant with small and medium sized organisations.

After reading and researching chemistry at Oxford, Tony Edwards joined the GKN Group as an operational research scientist. This lead to appointments in GKN Steel Company Ltd and from there, in 1968, into the re-nationalised, and subsequently privatised, British Steel plc. He has been a works manager and general manager of steelworks, a company director and served on the board of British Steel's Strip Products Division. He also worked for BSC (Industry) Ltd helping new businesses to set up in steel closure areas.

In 1991 Penarth Management invited Tony to join its team of consultants in order to develop its environmental consultancy expertise. Since its foundation in 1976, Penarth Management has specialised in working with smaller companies, a policy which leads to a continual search for simple uncomplicated management solutions and systems with the least amount of documentation. The fruits of this experience and approach are carried through into this book.

He is a registered environmental auditor with EARA (Environmental Auditors Registration Association), a Chartered Engineer and a Member of the Institute of Materials.

Chapter 1

Introduction to environmental management

What is environmental management?

What do we mean by the words 'environment' and 'environmental management'?

The word 'environment' is used in different ways. We talk of the 'home environment', the 'work environment', the 'social environment'. We use the word to describe our physical surroundings, made up of air, trees, grass. It is this latter use that is the subject of this book. Our concern must be for the world as a whole, its 'air, water, land, natural resources, flora, fauna, humans, and their inter-relations', to quote from ISO 14001.

By 'environmental management' we mean keeping control of our activities so that we do what we can to conserve these physical resources and to avoid polluting them. We can apply these controls in our life domestically, in what we buy and what we throw away, but it is usually in our work where the environmental impact of what we do is greatest. Such has been the impact of industrial activity that resources are becoming depleted and environmental damage is increasing. Some of the steps taken by the international community and governments to control and improve the situation are described in Chapter 2.

In this book, we are concerned with control at the level of the business, whether that be a chemical works or a refinery, engineering, printing, transport, or even office based businesses or teaching where the environmental impacts may be smaller but are still real. Because of the all-embracing nature of environmental management, the word 'organisation' has been used throughout the book to describe your business, firm or company.

What are the benefits?

There are four reasons why every organisation should take environmental factors into account in its management processes: ethical, economic, legal and commercial.

Ethical

As human beings we have a duty to look after the world in which we live and to hand it on to our children in good shape.

Economic

Conserving resources and not generating waste products or wasting energy means we save on cost.

There is also increasing evidence that insurance companies will consider a reduction in premiums if by having proper managerial control over environmental risks the likelihood of there being a disaster should be reduced. If your organisation is overseen by the

Environment Agency, i.e. your processes fall within the scope of the integrated pollution prevention and control legislation, it is heartening to note that the Agency is experimenting with linking the level of regulation to whether an organisation has an externally verified environmental management system or not.

Legal

More and more governments including our own are passing laws to control how we interact with the environment. Therefore we need systems to make sure we stay within the law, otherwise we can be fined and damage our reputation.

Commercial

More and more large organisations are taking control of their environmental responsibilities and they expect their suppliers and subcontractors to do the same. Without evidence of an environmental management system you may find the number of customers prepared to trade with you will start to fall. On the other hand, by being able to demonstrate good environmental practice, new market opportunities may open up to you.

ISO 14001

ISO 14001 has been developed as a formalised structure for an environmental management system which can be independently assessed for compliance. This corresponds exactly to the ISO 9001 quality systems which will be familiar to many readers. In fact, as is shown throughout the book, organisations that are already registered to ISO 9001 can integrate their environmental management system with their existing ISO 9001 structure and so build on what they already have rather than starting anew.

ISO 14001 can be adopted by any organisation. There are no restrictions on the type of activities which can be assessed. It is hoped that non-manufacturing organisations will read this book and decide that environmental management is as much for them as it is for the factory down the road.

What will it cost?

As with any management initiative, the biggest cost is the effort that you have to put into creating, launching and maintaining your environmental management system. This book is intended to help you to do this as painlessly as possible by leading you through each stage of the process and offering you sample documents and texts that you can adapt to fit your circumstances, instead of your having to start with a blank sheet of paper and wondering where to go next. The book is intended to be particularly helpful if you are a small organisation.

It is too easy to make things too complicated. The aim must be to create as simple a system as possible yet cover all the essentials. In this way you minimise the effort needed to create and maintain the system, you use less paper and you make it straightforward for your workforce to understand what is required of them. Success should be easier.

You cannot avoid the cost of the assessment, but by going into the market for competitive quotations you can be sure you are not paying too much. This is discussed further in Chapter 12.

Many organisations have found that they save more than the cost of the project in a year simply by giving attention to how they use energy in the forms of gas or electricity, or where they use water, or how much they are paying to dispose of the waste which they need not create.

This book

The book falls into four main sections:

- Chapters 2–4 describe the global environmental initiatives and the background to ISO 14001.
- Chapters 5–9 go through the stages of creating a documented environmental management system (EMS).

- Chapters 10–12 give advice on launching the EMS and how to prepare for the assessment.
- Chapters 13–14 describe the European Eco-Management & Audit Scheme (EMAS) and write about integrated management systems which can bring together environment, quality, health and safety, and other management functions.

The book is supported by three supplementary volumes which contain typical documents that you can use as models when you come to document your own environmental activities:

- model Registers of Environmental Aspects and Environmental Legislation;
- model Operating Procedures;
- model Environmental Management Manual.

These are also available on the accompanying website (see the Preface) and can be downloaded and adapted to suit your circumstances.

Chapter 2

The global perspective

The world's environment is continually changing. Originally this was caused by physical factors, for example erosion by rivers leading to mountains and valleys. Different forms of vegetation were caused by different climatic conditions depending on nearness to the equator. Cycles of long-term climate change led to glacial erosion followed by a return to warmer conditions; deserts were created by sun and wind.

Man has caused his own changes and in the last centuries, since the Industrial Revolution, the rate of change has become faster and faster. We need to use the world's resources to live and create all the things that we regard as necessary to live a good life. In the process we create pollutants and wastes that cause more and more damage and put the remaining resources at risk. For the sake of future generations some control has to be exercised.

Think for a moment of some of the biggest items which hit the news headlines fairly regularly. The holes in the ozone layer caused by volatile organic compounds reaching the stratosphere result in an increase in skin cancers. Greenhouse gases, particularly carbon dioxide from burning fuels and car exhausts and methane generated in rubbish tips will cause the temperature of the earth to rise, with potentially catastrophic results if the ice caps melt and sea levels rise. These are truly global in that the whole world contributes to the problem to a greater or lesser degree and the whole world has to find the solution. On the other hand there are more localised incidents that cause widespread and long term environmental damage. Being local and therefore subject to local decision making, one would have hoped that they should have been avoidable.

Consider Chernobyl, where substantial tracts of Belarus are still contaminated with radiation and children born since the explosion still die of radiation-induced diseases. More recently, there was the incident off north-west Spain in November 2002 when the tanker *Prestige* with 70 000 tonnes of oil on board broke up. Storms blew the oil onto the coast, spelling severe economic hardship for the Galician fishing villages and killing seabirds, fish and shellfish. The international dimensions of the incident are shown by the number of countries somehow involved: the *Prestige* was built in Japan, last inspected in Holland and owned by a Greek-controlled company registered in Liberia. The tanker was registered in the Bahamas with a Greek captain, a Filipino crew and chartered by a Russian company to carry oil loaded in Latvia to Singapore.

These were large well publicised events. The technical press regularly contains accounts of smaller misdemeanours which lead to environmental damage (and resultant fines by the courts). Some of these also have long term effects, such as the pollution of ground water making it unfit for human consumption.

International and governmental action

The serious threats to our environment have been increasingly recognised by governments since the 1960s, gathering momentum all the time. Some of the landmark milestones at the international level are described in the following paragraphs.

The Brundtland Report 1987

The World Commission on Environment and Development chaired by Norway's Prime Minister Gro Harlem Brundtland produced a report 'Our Common Future'. In it, the phrase 'sustainable development' was defined as 'forms of progress which meet the needs of the present without compromising the ability of future generations to meet their own needs'.

Montreal Protocol on Substances that Deplete the Ozone Layer 1987

In particular, this protocol led to the phasing out of chlorofluorocarbons (CFCs) as propellants in aerosols, as foaming agents in fire extinguishers and as refrigerants. The protocol has been regularly strengthened in the succeeding ten years.

United Nations Conference on Environment and Development 1992 ('Earth Summit')

The Rio de Janeiro conference in 1992 issued a declaration which included calling on national governments to 'enact legislation and to formulate plans at national and local level to promote improved air quality, protect the quality of the environment and land-based resources, and address the problems of waste, poverty and lifestyles, and disseminate environmentally sound technology'. Another important outcome was a broad agreement requiring industrial countries to reduce emissions to 1990 levels by 2000.

The UN Framework Convention on Climate Change 1997

The UN's concern for climate change took a further significant step with the Kyoto Protocol, which set the target of reducing the emission of greenhouse gases to 5.2 per cent below 1990 levels by 2008–2012.

World Summit on Sustainable Development 2002 ('Second Earth Summit')

The Johannesburg conference was billed as Rio + 10. Reactions to the outcome of the conference were mixed, with some people feeling that hard progress was obscured by politics. Nevertheless, firm commitments were agreed, including:

- harmonising the classification of chemicals by 2008 and producing and using chemicals that will not harm human health by 2020;
- increasing the efficient use of energy and the proportion of energy from renewable sources;
- reversing the trend of losses in biodiversity by 2010;
- ending destructive fishing and establishing protected areas by 2012.

Ongoing actions

Concern for the environment is an ongoing concern, which is reflected in the ever increasing body of legislation. Some of this is in response to international pressures, some to European pressures, as well as originating with the government of the UK. A few examples are:

- Finance Bills (Budgets) – company cars taxed according to emissions, climate change levy (energy tax).
- Landfill tax – to discourage landfilling.
- Pollution Prevention and Control Act 1999 – emissions and effluents from industrial processes.
- Water Industry Act 1991 and Waste Resources Act 1991 – pollution of water.
- Producer Responsibility Obligations (Packaging Waste) Regulations 1997 – to minimise packaging and promote recycling.
- The Landfill Regulations 2002 – to stop co-disposal of hazardous and non-hazardous waste.

Soon, the above will be followed by:

- the forthcoming adoption of the End-of-Life Vehicles Directive and the Waste Electrical and Electronic Equipment Directive into UK law – to promote recycling.

A comprehensive overview

The key indicators of environmental impact that need to be at the front of every person's mind when planning any change, and the types of actions that cause that impact, are shown in the following tables:

Climate change

Effect	Examples of causes
Global warming	Vehicle exhaust emissions, power station and furnace emissions.
Ozone depletion	Use of CFCs (now banned).
Deforestation	Logging; burning forest for short-term agricultural gain.
Acid rain	Power station emissions e.g. SO_2 and NOx.
Desertification	Over extraction of natural water supplies; removing vegetation, trees, hedges.

Pollution

Effect	Examples of causes
Air pollution	Gaseous emissions from factories, vehicles.
Water pollution	Chemical discharges to drains and watercourses.
Land contamination	Toxic substances disposed of incorrectly; spillages.

Natural resources

Resource	Examples of how the resource is depleted
Fuels	Burning of fossil fuels e.g. coal, oil, gas; wasting energy.
Land	Landfill; erosion; building.
Water	Over-extraction; pollution of natural water sources.
Minerals	Over-extraction.
Clean air	Emissions; vehicle exhausts.
Biodiversity	Poor farming practices e.g. monoculture, use of pesticides and herbicides; destruction of habitats and sites of special scientific interest (SSSIs).
Waste hierarchy	Little attempt to move up the waste hierarchy from landfill (least desirable); incinerate for energy; re-use; recycle; reduce (best option).

Benefits

Resource	Examples of action
Energy	Insulate buildings; switch off lights and computers; buy energy efficient equipment.
Resources	Economical use of resources reduces costs.
Waste	Producing less waste saves resources and reduces disposal costs.
Marketing	Reductions in costs lead to more competitively priced products; consumers and customers are becoming more environmentally aware.

The waste hierarchy

Whilst the elimination of waste completely brings many advantages, not least the savings of the cost of the wasted materials purchased and the cost of the labour and machines used to convert them into your product, as well as reducing the cost of disposing of the waste, it is not always possible to achieve this desirable outcome.

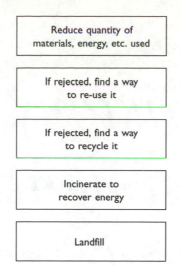

Fig. 2.1 The waste hierarchy

There are steps along the way which are shown in the waste hierarchy in Fig. 2.1, starting with the most desirable outcome at the top, down to the least desirable outcome at the bottom. Any improvement which lifts a waste product higher up the list is welcome.

Environmental management systems

By deciding to create an environmental management system and work for registration to ISO 14001, your organisation is saying to the world that you care about all the above issues and are determined to play your part in making sure that the world can continue to sustain our civilisation into future generations.

Chapter 3
Brief history of environmental standards

BS 7750

Although particular aspects of environmental control had been the subject of legislation in past decades, for example the Control of Pollution Act 1974 and the Trade Effluent Regulations 1989, it was the Environmental Protection Act 1990 which significantly raised the profile of the environment as an industrial responsibility and which brought many industrial activities under the direct control of the Environment Agency or the local authorities. Organisations needed to put systems in place to ensure that they complied with the terms of their licences. The growing international concerns about environmental sustainability added to the pressures. The success of the quality management standard BS 5750 (as ISO 9001 was then known in the UK) gave a model for a management system. So the idea of an environmental management was born. BSI's choice of the reference number BS 7750 clearly showed the intention to ally the new standard to the earlier one.

BS 7750 was first published in 1992. To ensure that it was a workable and an effective standard the next 12 months were used to run pilot schemes with organisations representing some 40 sectoral groups ranging from engineering or timber trades to the food industry and agriculture. This experience led to revisions and the first general version of the standard was published in 1994. By 1995 certification bodies had been accredited to assess to the new standard and the first certificates were awarded.

EMAS

Running alongside this activity was the European Commission's initiative, the Eco-Management and Auditing Scheme (EMAS), which came into force in 1995 and which has a considerable overlap with ISO 14001. This is described in more detail in Chapter 13.

ISO 14001

The International Standards Organisation recognised the need for an international standard for environmental management. In the same way as the international quality standard ISO 9000 was based on BS 5750, so ISO 14001 grew out of BS 7750. It was published in 1996, leading to the withdrawal of BS 7750.

ISO 14001 has now been in existence for some years. Under the rules governing the updating of standards, the process of review and revision is underway. The revised Standard is due to be published in 2004–2005; the early indications are that the changes are designed to give greater clarity to the requirements of the Standard as it exists now rather than being a fundamental review. However, even when published, organisations that are already certified will be given a substantial time period in which to incorporate the changes into their existing EMS. If the change from ISO 9001: 1994 to ISO 9001: 2000 is a guide, the time period could be as long as three years.

Therefore, if you decide to start work on preparing for assessment to ISO 14001 now, you can have confidence that what you do will be stable for some years to come.

Chapter 4
Introduction to ISO 14001

Introduction

In this chapter we take a general look at the content of ISO 14001 and its requirements. The detailed study of the requirements and how to put them into practice comes in Chapters 6, 7 and 8.

ISO 14001 is not an isolated standard. It is part of a family of supporting standards, details of which are included in this chapter.

Finally, there is a comparison of the structure of ISO 14001 and ISO 9001: 2000, where it becomes apparent that there are considerable similarities, particularly in the way that the different management systems are controlled. This gives an opportunity for organisations that are already registered to ISO 9001 to integrate their quality and environmental systems.

The clauses of ISO 14001

The following synopsis of ISO 14001 gives a quick understanding of the range of standard's requirements. It is no substitute for looking at the full text of the standard. Your assessor will expect you to have a copy and you should purchase one. Standards are obtainable in the UK from the British Standards Institution. The address for sales is given in Appendix D.

The requirements for environmental management systems are set out in Clause 4 of the Standard under six main headings:

4.1   General requirements
4.2   Environmental policy
4.3   Planning
4.4   Implementation and operations
4.5   Checking and corrective action
4.6   Management review

These are then when necessary divided into sub-clauses.

4.1 General requirements

There must be a documented environmental management system (EMS) that meets all the following requirements.

4.2 Environmental policy

There must be an environmental policy that is consistent with any group or sector policy, is relevant to the organisation's activities, commits to prevent pollution and observe relevant legislation, has a commitment to continual improvement and setting environmental objectives and targets, and states how it is made available to all employees and publicly.

4.3 Planning

4.3.1 Environmental aspects

Environmental aspects shall be identified both for normal operating conditions, for reasonably foreseeable deviations and for emergencies. This is usually documented in a Register of Environmental Aspects.

4.3.2 Legal and other requirements

Relevant legislative, regulatory and other environmental requirements must be identified. This is usually documented in a Register of Environmental Legislation which must be kept up to date.

4.3.3 Objectives and targets

Environmental improvement objectives and targets must be set, consistent with the policy.

4.3.4 Environmental management programme

Programmes must be set for the achievement of the objectives and targets, and responsibilities must be designated.

4.4 Implementation and operation

4.4.1 Structure and responsibility

Responsibilities must be defined. Adequate human resources with appropriate skills must be provided. There must be a management representative with the authority to ensure the EMS is implemented and to make sure that performance is reported upon to management.

4.4.2 Training, awareness and competence

All employees must be aware of the environmental objectives, have appropriate job training in relevant environmental procedures and know the consequences of departing from the procedures.

4.4.3 Communication

There must be a system for receiving and responding to communications regarding environmental aspects, from both external and internal sources.

4.4.4 Environmental management system and documentation

There must be a documented description of the environmental management system, which brings together the policy, objectives and targets, and responsibilities. It must point to all the associated documentation (e.g. the Registers, Operating Procedures, including emergency plans).

4.4.5 Document control

There must be a system for document control.

4.4.6 Operational control

Documented procedures and Work Istructions must be prepared where they are needed to ensure compliance with the requirements of the EMS. These should also relate to goods and services with significant environmental aspects, and be communicated to suppliers and contractors. For example, when contractors are working on site, whether in a long-term or short-term capacity, they need to be aware of, and observe, the local environmental rules and procedures. Assessors are paying particular attention to the control of contractors, simply because experience has shown that they can be the cause of a significant number of environmental incidents. Going one stage further, although not a specific requirement of ISO 14001, good environmental practice suggests that enquiries should be made about the environmental status or performance of key suppliers and subcontractors.

4.4.7 Emergency preparedness and response

Reasonably foreseeable and emergency situations must be identified and appropria procedures implemented. They must be reviewed, especially if they have ever been calle into action, and tested periodically.

4.5 Checking and corrective action

4.5.1 Monitoring and measurement

There must be procedures for monitoring activities which impact on the environment. Any monitoring equipment must be calibrated.

4.5.2 Nonconformance and corrective and preventive action

There must be a system for handling noncompliances, with investigation and corrective actions.

4.5.3 Environmental management records

Records must be kept and archiving requirements specified.

4.5.4 Environmental management system audit

The EMS must be audited regularly to ensure the system is operating effectively. There must be an audit programme and a reporting and follow-up system.

4.6 Management review

Management must periodically review the environmental policy, objectives and the EMS to ensure they are still effective and relevant to the organisation's needs in the light of changing circumstances.

Annex A and ISO 14004

The standard contains an Annex A giving very useful guidance and additional information on the interpretation of the standard.

This is further supplemented by ISO 14004 'Environmental management systems – General guidelines on principles, systems and supporting techniques'. This is particularly helpful when writing about the benefits of having an EMS and when preparing to carry out an initial environmental review, and at the planning stage of the project.

The structure of the documented environmental management system

The structure of the final documented EMS will be as shown in Fig. 4.1.

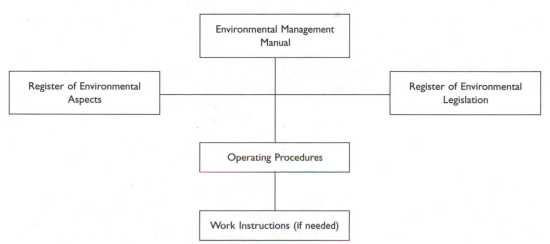

Fig. 4.1 The structure of a documented environmental management system

Table 4.1

ISO 14001 : 1996	Environmental management systems – Specification with guidance for use
ISO 14004 : 1996	Environmental management systems – General guidelines on principles, systems and supporting techniques
ISO 14015 : 2001	Environmental assessment of sites and organisations
ISO 14020 series	Environmental labels and labelling (published in 1999 and 2000)
ISO 14031 : 2000	Environmental performance evaluation – Guidelines
DD ISO/TR 14032:2000	Examples of environmental performance evaluation
ISO 14040 : 1997	Environmental management – Life cycle assessment – Principles and framework
ISO 14041 : 1998	Environmental management – Life cycle assessment – Goal and scope definition and inventory analysis
ISO 14042 : 2000	Environmental management – Life cycle assessment – Impact assessment
ISO 14043 : 2000	Environmental management – Life cycle assessment – Interpretation
DD ISO/TS 14048 : 2002	Life cycle assessment – Data documentation format
PD ISO/TR 14049 : 2002	Examples of application of ISO 14041 to goal and scope definition and inventory analysis
ISO 14050 : 2002	Environmental management – Vocabulary
ISO 19011 : 2002	Guidelines for quality and/or environmental management systems auditing

The ISO 14000 family

The International Standards Organisation (ISO) attaches such importance to the development of environmental management standards that it has allocated the range of numbers 14000–14099 to environmental topics. A number of the standards have already been published and others are in the course of preparation. The most significant ones are included in Table 4.1. These standards have been adopted by the British Standards Institution, and are mostly prefixed BS in the UK.

However, in the first instance concentrate on ISO 14001, and as suggested above, you may also find ISO 14004 helpful.

Similarities with ISO 9001

In writing this book, I have assumed that the organisation may wish to create a free-standing environmental management system, i.e. registration to ISO 9001 is not a prerequisite for going forward to ISO 14001. However, the job will be that much easier if a quality management system already exists. The possibility of having common Operating Procedures for both management systems is recognised in the model Operating Procedures.

The overlap between ISO 14001 and ISO 9001: 2000 is shown in Table 4.2. Where bold text has been used, it should be possible to write an Operating Procedure which is common to both the environmental and quality management systems.

Table 4.2 Similarities between ISO 14001 and ISO 9001: 2000

ISO 14001		ISO 9001: 2000	
Clause no		**Clause no**	
4.1	Environmental management system	4.1	Quality management system – General requirements
4.2	Environmental policy	5.3	Quality policy
4.3.3	Objectives and targets	5.4.1	Quality objectives
4.3.4	Environmental management programme	5.4.2	Quality management system planning
4.4.1	Structure and responsibility	5.5.1	Responsibility and authority
		5.5.2	Management representative
4.4.2	**Training, awareness and competence**	6.2.2	**Competence, awareness and training**
4.4.3	**Communication**	5.5.3	**Internal communication**
4.4.4	Environmental management system and documentation	4.2.1	Documentation requirements – general
4.4.5	**Document control**	4.2.3	**Control of documents**
4.4.6	Operational control	7.5.1	Control of production and service provision
4.5.1	**Monitoring and measurement**	7.6	**Control of monitoring and measuring devices**
4.5.2	**Non-conformance and corrective and preventive action**	8.3	Control of non-conforming product
		8.5.2	Corrective action
		8.5.3	**Preventive action**
4.5.3	**Environmental management records**	4.2.4	**Control of quality records**
4.5.4	**Environmental management system audit**	8.2.2	**Internal audit**
4.6	Management review	5.6	Management review

Chapter 5
Planning the project

Introduction

The logic of ISO 14001 is illustrated in Fig. 5.1. In this chapter we consider how to follow the logic, by creating a programme that will lead from the initial decision to create an environmental management system to a successful assessment to ISO 14001.

The programme falls into 11 steps, as follows:

- commitment
- resources
- communication
- environmental legislation and environmental aspects

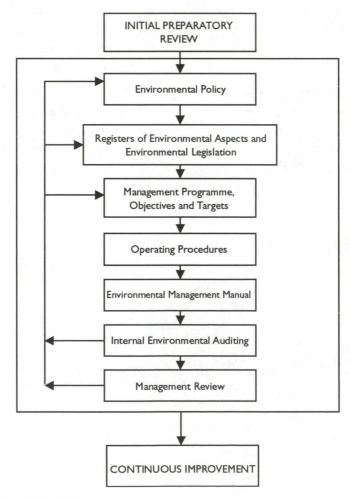

Fig. 5.1 The logic of ISO 14001

- management objectives and policy
- procedures
- writing the manual
- implementation
- auditing
- choosing your assessor
- assessment

Step 1: Commitment

Unless there is full commitment from the top to the bottom of the organisation, the process of creating and implementing your environmental management system and then going forward for assessment will be difficult, or could even fail. Even if you are ultimately successful, the timetable will become so drawn out that people will lose interest.

Clause 4.2 of the Standard requires the organisation to have an environmental policy, but it is difficult to write a policy in sufficient detail until some of the work, e.g. defining the environmental aspects, has been carried out. So, in order to set the process in motion, a statement of intent should be written and well publicised. This should be signed by the chairman, managing director, chief executive, general manager, or whoever is the top person at the site involved. It would be even better if the members of the board, or the senior managers, all signed the statement.

Suitable wording is shown in Fig. 5.2.

This statement of intent will be replaced by the environmental policy later in the project (see Step 5).

ENVIRONMENTAL STATEMENT OF INTENT

.... Limited is a company which cares about the environment.

We will comply with all relevant environmental legislation.

We will define the impacts which our operations have on the environment. We will promote good environmental practice, and eliminate or reduce bad impacts.

To help us achieve our aim, we will create an environmental management system which satisfies the requirements of BS EN ISO 14001, and will seek assessment and formal registration to the Standard.

All managers and employees are committed to this process, which will also involve our suppliers and subcontractors.

....
Managing Director   Sales Director

....
Works Manager   Chief Accountant

....
Personnel Manager   Technical Manager

[date]

Fig. 5.2

Step 2: Resources

Decide who is going to drive the project for the organisation. This needs to be someone who is well respected and has the authority to take and implement decisions. He or she also needs an orderly mind, and ideally will have direct access to the managing director or top person.

This person has been called the environmental manager in this book. In much of the literature about environmental management, the title 'environmental champion' is used. This certainly describes the sort of person who is needed to carry out this role.

In many companies with an established quality system the quality manager is able to take on the environmental job. Some companies prefer to ally it to health and safety. Others pick a separate individual.

Because of the overlap between the different management systems – the overlap with ISO 9001 is described in Chapter 4 – the managers responsible for different systems need to be able to work together.

Then decide whether your environmental manager needs extra help either from within or outside the organisation. The latter can be in the form of outside specialist environmental consultants, though this book is intended to act as your personal consultant. A note on choosing consultants is included at the end of this chapter.

For example, once the need has been found for a written procedure, why not ask the person who is already doing the job to write down how it is done? The environmental manager then has three tasks:

- Check that the procedure is comprehensive, and meets the requirements of the Standard.
- Put the text into the standard format.
- Have the procedure authorised and issued.

Tell everybody the name of the person who will be driving the project when you have your communication sessions.

Step 3: Communication

Before pinning the statement on the notice board, the decision to create an environmental management system should be explained to everybody. Communication throughout the organisation at certain key stages in the programme is essential if each person is to play their part. These communication points are detailed in the programme described in this chapter.

How communication is carried out will depend on the size of the organisation and how it is structured. Sometimes it is feasible for the managing director to talk to everybody, either all together or in groups. Otherwise, managers will need to be briefed to pass the message down, maybe to their foremen/supervisors who will speak to the rest of the employees. If you have a tradition of 'toolbox talks', i.e. 10 minute sessions with each team at their place of work, then use one of these to explain the commitment.

As explained in Step 1, everyone must be involved. For example, it is only too apparent when reading accounts of court cases where companies are accused of causing pollution that the fault often lies with a particular individual who might be quite low down in the organisation who did not understand the importance of his or her job in preserving the environment.

It is a good idea to produce a simple briefing note as an aide-memoire to the speakers. An outline briefing note is included in Appendix A.

At these sessions, always try to involve the audience. If you use them as an occasion simply to deliver the message from 'on high' with no opportunity for feedback you will not create a sense of involvement. Invite people to identify a few of the environmental aspects which are relevant to them or to the organisation as a whole. Get them to explain whether they have ways of controlling them. If they have, ask whether they are written down so that anyone can know how to handle the aspect correctly? You may be taken by surprise at the concern for the environment shown by much of the population at large. This particularly applies to young people. Tap into this enthusiasm.

Step 4: Environmental aspects and legislation

The first step towards creating a management system is to find out your starting position, both in terms of the environmental impacts caused by your activities and the legislation which the organisation has to observe. Although ISO 14001 does not state that you *must* carry out an initial review, it is obviously sensible to do one in a systematic way. ISO 14004, the guideline document, clause 4.1.3, talks about establishing the current position by means of an initial environmental review, and lists topics which can be considered.

Chapter 6 describes how to tackle this stage of the project, and how to record and evaluate the information you collect, by compiling the Register of Environmental Aspects and the Register of Environmental Legislation.

This is not a stage to be hurried. It is truly said that a firm structure can only be built on strong foundations. Finding out which statutory regulations apply to your organisation, and which activities impact on the environment and how big the impacts are, needs a careful study.

Step 5: Management objectives

A key feature of the Standard is the word 'improvement'. The concept of improvement is now also a part of the revised ISO 9001:2000 Quality Standard. Assessors regularly look for evidence of improvement objectives and progress.

Your first objective will be to obey the law. Then, once you know what your impacts are, you will be able to decide where improvements need to be, or can be, made. This will need top management discussion, but taking these decisions should not be difficult. A systematic way of evaluating the relative importance of environmental aspects is described in Chapter 6.

Once all this is known, the time has come to rewrite the environmental policy. No longer is it a statement of intent. You know what your impacts are, you know what your objectives are. It is now for real. Chapter 6 will help you to write your policy.

Step 6: Procedures

With the list of relevant legislation and a list of aspects and management objectives available, the titles of the procedures you need will start to become apparent. For example, procedures may be required:

- to make sure that you keep within the law;
- to provide any data required by a regulatory body, e.g. the Local Authority, the Environment Agency;
- to keep the impacts under control;
- to keep particular processes under control;
- to handle emergencies.

You will probably find that the people directly responsible already have ways of working, which may or may not be documented, to keep control of the situation. They will all need to be put into your standard format, and checked to make sure they are sufficiently comprehensive and meet all the requirements of the Standard.

Chapter 7 explains which procedures might be needed, and gives help and practical examples on how to write them.

Writing, issuing and checking the procedures can be quite a long process. To make it as painless and as effective as possible, they should be tackled in a systematic way and issued, in draft, *as you go along*. In this way, they are introduced in bite-sized instalments and can be assimilated more easily.

Some people feel they should wait until *all* the procedures are written before they have a grand 'launching' event. First of all, this wastes valuable implementation and training time. Second, it gives people mental indigestion. Third, at worst, it is viewed as the imposition of extra bureaucracy and something to be resisted. This does not mean you do not eventually have a grand launch. This is still desirable and comes along in Step 8.

Step 7: Writing the manual

At this point in the programme it should be possible to pull together all the work done so far into the Environmental Management Manual.

The manual describes how the business meets the requirements of each clause and subclause of the Standard. It will start with the policy, and describe all the component parts of the management system. It will describe how you manage and keep up to date the Registers of Environmental Legislation and Environmental Aspects, how you set objectives, organisation and training, the procedures, how you react when things go wrong and how you put them right, how you monitor the system to make sure it is behaving properly and keep it up to date, and how the management reviews and controls the whole process.

Chapter 9 gives detailed guidance on writing the manual.

Step 8: Launching the system

Having created your environmental management system (EMS) on paper, it has to be put into practice. The stages of launching the system are:

- The first formal environmental management review meeting – to approve and adopt the EMS and plan the next stages of the project. This also sets the date when the EMS officially came into being.
- Planning document distribution.
- Communication – now is the time to carry out your next communication exercise so that everybody knows what is happening and the plans for the future.
- Training – it is quite possible that certain people will need some specific training. This needs to be carried out now.

Chapter 10 explains the launch process in more detail.

Step 9: Auditing

You need to decide who are going to be your internal environmental auditors.
Chapter 11 gives guidance on:

- choosing your auditors;
- training your auditors;
- managing and carrying out audits;
- reporting, corrective actions and follow-up.

The whole EMS, which means every clause of the manual, every procedure and any associated Work Instructions, has to be checked to make sure that it has been correctly implemented.

As your auditors will probably still be doing their normal jobs as well as taking on auditing, and also bearing in mind that the people being audited still have a job to do and cannot keep on stopping to attend to an auditor, this stage of the project needs careful planning. How long the overall auditing programme will take will depend on the size of the business, the number of procedures, and how much time people can devote to it.

One thing is certain. You must not let the difficulties described above distract you into letting the programme become too drawn out. You need to make an impact and create an impetus that will carry you through to the assessment.

This is discussed in more detail in Chapter 11, but for the sake of argument a period of three months has been allowed in the timetable shown in Fig. 5.3.

The first round of audits will inevitably find weaknesses in the procedures and many of them will need to be revised and reissued, and then re-audited.

You will also find places in the business where the procedures are satisfactory but are not being observed. Again, a re-audit will be required.

Step 10: Choosing your assessor

The assessment bodies are busy. You need to choose your assessor at least five months before the date you are planning for your final assessment.

Chapter 12 deals with the process of choosing your assessor in some detail.

If you are already registered to ISO 9001, you will probably find that your quality assessment body is also accredited by UKAS to carry out ISO 14001 assessments, and they will obviously be keen to have this extra business. So, always ask your existing assessment body for a quotation. But it would be worthwhile seeking other quotations. You might be tempted to put all your business elsewhere if your existing assessor becomes too uncompetitive.

Note the recommendation in Chapter 12 that you should choose a certification body that will give you a pre-audit visit. This is even more important in the case of environmental management than in quality management, because the assessor will come to a conclusion about whether or not the scope of your EMS is comprehensive before the final day of reckoning. It is possible to overlook a particular but important item of legislation or aspect, or to have inadequate controls. These will be picked up early on and you can plug the gaps. If this were to be left to the assessment proper, a serious non-compliance would arise and you would fail.

You can arrange your pre-visit any time after you have launched your EMS, and it needs to be 6–8 weeks before your final assessment.

Step 11: Assessment

You have:

- chosen your assessor;
- had your pre-audit visit and made any subsequent corrections to the documented EMS;
- audited your complete environmental management system;
- revised the system and reaudited where necessary.

The day of the assessment is approaching. Chapter 12 describes the actions and checks that you need to take to make sure that everything goes smoothly. This includes telling everybody what to expect when the assessor arrives to talk to them, and how they should respond and behave.

The overall programme and timetable

We can now put all the steps together and produce an overall programme and timetable. How long will it all take?

A realistic time-scale is shown in Fig. 5.3. It shows that the time-consuming steps are:

- carrying out the review which leads to the completion of the Register of Environmental Legislation and the Register of Environmental Aspects;
- writing procedures;
- auditing and revising procedures.

The 10 month time-scale from a standing start to assessment is quite feasible for a business of 40–100 employees. Smaller businesses might save up to two months.

With larger businesses, it all becomes a matter of resources. Once the review has been completed and the objectives set, the amount of work required to write procedures and audit them should become apparent. With sufficient resources, there is no reason why the overall 10 months should not be achieved. What is important is that sufficient resources are made available to keep the project moving, whether provided internally or with some external help. If the project is not to lose its momentum with the risk of boredom setting in, no timetable should be allowed which exceeds 15 months overall.

Fig. 5.3 The timetable

Step No	Activity	Jan	Feb	Mar	Apr	May	Jun	Jul	Aug	Sep	Oct	Nov
1	Commitment	*										
2	Resources	* *										
3	Communication	*	*									
4	Define legislation & aspects		* * *	* * *								
5	Management objectives & policy				* *							
6	Write and issue draft procedures and work instructions				* * *	* * *						
7	Write manual						* *					
8	Implement											
	– management meeting						*					
	– launch						*	*				
9	Auditing											
	– train auditors					* *	* *					
	– auditing							* *	* * * * * *	* * *		
	– revise procedures							* *	* * * * * *	* * *	*	
10	Choose assessor				* * * *							
11	Assessment											
	– pre-visit							*				
	– preparation									* *	* *	
	– assessment										*	
	– registration											*

Customer concerns

In the same way that, in the late 1980s and early 1990s, many major companies started to require their suppliers and subcontractors to be registered to ISO 9001, so today they are equally concerned about environmental performance.

QS 9000

One expression of this is in the QS 9000 standard compiled by Chrysler, Ford, General Motors and other vehicle manufacturers to apply the principles of ISO 9001 to automotive suppliers and subcontractors, and which includes the words under Clause 4.9 'A supplier shall have a process to ensure compliance with all applicable government safety and environmental regulations, including those concerning handling, recycling, eliminating or disposing of hazardous materials. This should be evidenced by appropriate certificates or letters of compliance.' Obviously, registration to ISO 14001 satisfies this requirement.

Land Rover

As an example of a another company with environmental concerns, Land Rover set environmental milestones for its suppliers and subcontractors, and asked for a commitment and a timetable for each step. As would be expected, these parallel the steps described in this chapter, as can be seen from the example in Fig. 5.4.

This is one example of how a major business addresses its environmental responsibilities. There are, and will be many more. By taking the decision to work for ISO 14001 and approaching the work in a structured way, you will be able to convince your customers, should they ask, that you know what you are doing.

Other programmes

Project Acorn and BS 8555

Project Acorn was a pilot study being run jointly by BSI and the Department of the Environment, Transport and the Regions (DETR) started in mid 2000 involving some large companies and their suppliers. It is similar to the Land Rover approach and is based on a

		Plan date	Achievement date
Milestone 1	Management commitment		
Milestone 2	Environmental impact assessment		
Milestone 3	Identify legislation		
Milestone 4	Environmental effects register		
Milestone 5	Environmental policy		
Milestone 6	Environmental strategy key goals and targets		
Milestone 7	Develop action plan		
Milestone 8	Implementation of an environmental management system		
Milestone 9	Audit system		
Milestone 10	EMAS or ISO 14001		

Fig. 5.4 Land Rover's environmental milestones

Phase	Title	Content
1	Commitment and baseline review.	Top management's public commitment. Identify the organisation's significant environmental aspects.
2	Identify and ensure compliance with relevant environmental law and other relevant charters or codes of practice.	Prepare the Register of Environmental Legislation and check compliance.
3	Develop objectives, targets and management programme, e.g. procedures.	Finalise environmental policy. Set objectives and targets. Write procedures to control aspects, ensure compliance and achieve targets.
4	Implementation and operation.	Training. Implement procedures.
5	Checking	Auditing, corrective action, review.
6	Final assessment	

Fig. 5.5 BS 8555

model originally developed by the Irish Productivity Centre, Dublin. The results of the study are being formalised into BS 8555 'Guide to the phased implementation of an environmental management system', to be published in 2003. The creation and implementation of an EMS is divided into six phases as shown in Fig. 5.5. Each phase can be assessed as it is completed, which should make the final assessment an easier process.

Conclusion

Remember, though, that the real reason for creating an environmental management system is so that you:

- stay within the law;
- know what impact your activities have on the environment;
- take active steps to reduce your impacts;
- take the benefit of the savings you will make, as well as
- satisfying your customers.

This chapter has set out to describe the steps needed to create and implement an environmental management system that can be successfully assessed to ISO 14001.

Chapters 6–8 work through the requirements of the Standard, clause by clause, and give detailed advice on how to tackle each one.

Using consultants

Even though this book is intended to act as your personal guide to the project, you may decide you would like some help from outside. This usually comes in the shape of a consultant.

Consultants can do all or some of the following work for you:

- Carry out the initial review.
- Write your Registers.
- Steer you through the objectives and target setting phase.
- Write your Operating Procedures.
- Write your Manual.
- Help you launch the EMS.
- Make periodic visits to check what you have done and give advice on any difficulties.
- Train internal environmental auditors, or convert your quality auditors into environmental auditors.

- Carry out a dummy assessment in advance of the real assessment.
- Help you maintain the EMS.

So how to choose a consultant? Recommendation by word of mouth from someone you trust is the best way. Another source can be your local Business Link or TEC who will have a list of consultants approved by them. Full members and associates of the Institute of Environmental Management and Assessment (IEMA), whose address is in Appendix D, will have had to demonstrate their competence in environmental management and assessment. The IEMA also registers environmental auditors through the Environmental Auditor's Registration Association (EARA).

Interview your prospective consultants. You will only be building up trouble for yourself if you engage someone, no matter how good they are, if the 'chemistry' between you both does not work. Find out what sorts of organisations they have worked for; ring some of them up and ask for a reference. Are these organisations similar to you in size and is the expertise transferable to your type of organisation? There have been instances of consultancy not working because the consultants carried 'big firm' experience, which tends to be more bureaucratic, into a small organisation. Get the consultants to show you the type of documentation they are used to creating. Make sure the consultant you see is the consultant who will actually do the work. See more than one consultant and compare quotations, but do remember that the cheapest may not be the best.

A fee rate of £250 to £550 per day including expenses would be reasonable. The number of days depends on how much work you want the consultant to do. If you want everything from the initial review through writing the documentation and internal auditing to assessment, think in terms of 12 to 15 days for an organisation of 50 employees with no 'nasty' environmental processes. When interviewing prospective consultants, always ask whether any grants are available. There are many incentives available to help improve environmental performance, for example from Business Links, and any good consultant will know what is on offer and whether you might qualify for some of it. The consultant's bill to you might be halved as a result.

Chapter 6
Policy and planning

Environmental policy (ISO 14001 Clause 4.2)

ISO 14001 Clause 4.2 requires the organisation to write and publicise an environmental policy, and is quite specific about what the policy must include:

- a commitment to continual improvement;
- a commitment to prevent pollution;
- a commitment to comply with relevant environmental regulations and any requirements such as an industry sector code of practice or the policy of a parent company;
- a commitment to set and progress objectives and targets;
- a statement that the environmental management system (EMS) is documented, implemented and maintained;
- a statement that the policy has been communicated to all employees;
- a statement that the policy is available to the public.

In addition, you may wish to introduce other ideas. For example, you may have a policy of active involvement in environmental issues in the local community; you may have developed life cycle assessment for your products; you may wish to highlight your intentions to reduce energy usage; you may have a land clean-up initiative.

The policy must be appropriate to the nature of your business. It is not uncommon for assessors to find policies which have obviously been borrowed from some other type of industrial sector without due thought. As an example, the following phrases found in the environmental policy of an educational establishment do not quite ring true – 'will make us a better company', 'compliance with licence requirements'.

It is for this reason that Chapter 5 advocates a two-stage process. Write an Environmental Statement of Intent at the beginning of the project. Then write the policy once the environmental status of the organisation is fully understood, i.e. when the initial review has been completed, the key environmental aspects have been defined and the first set of management objectives have been agreed.

A model policy is shown at the beginning of the model Environmental Management Manual. In writing this model, the mandatory elements have all been included, together with a few optional items. It is the optional items which make the policy real for your organisation. Otherwise the policy looks like something that has been bought off-the-shelf and will have less impact.

The policy needs to make an impact both visually and in what it says. It should be contained within a well laid out single page of A4 paper. It should be signed by the chief executive, or even all the members of the board or the senior managers. The wording needs to be kept short and straightforward, so that even the least able of readers understands what it means.

As the policy has to be communicated to all employees, the simplest way is to display well laid out copies on key noticeboards including your reception area. It is worthwhile spending £10 on a decent frame. It will give the policy importance (and it is less likely to be defaced). The policy can also be reproduced in company statements, e.g. the annual report.

The starting position (Step 4)

ISO 14001 Clause 4.3 requires you to define your environmental aspects, state which regulations have to be observed, and to define aims and objectives for improvement.

The only way to establish your starting position is to carry out an initial environmental review. If the review is properly comprehensive, by the end you will have defined:

- environmental aspects;
- relevant regulations;
- what environmental procedures or Work Instructions you already have in place, even though they might not have been recognised as such;
- whether you have any environmental trouble spots;
- where you have the opportunity to improve performance or make savings.

Carrying out the environmental review

You have to decide whether to carry out the review yourself using people within your organisation, or whether to use an external person. There is a good case for involving an outsider. None of us see all our own problems because we are too used to living with them, particularly if they have been around for years. The outsider can be a consultant, or you might find that a friendly major customer would be willing to lend you an expert for a couple of days to amplify your own efforts. Chapter 5 gives advice on how to find a suitable consultant.

If you are going to do the work yourself you need more than one person, drawn from different disciplines, e.g. production and administration, to prevent any predetermined ideas that will lead to a blinkered approach. You need people who have a fairly good overview of your activities, and who will be respected by the rest of the workforce. The next sections of the chapter give you guidance on how to proceed.

Environmental aspects (Clause 4.3.1)

Defining the environmental aspects

Your team can make a good start by remembering that impact on the environment largely means impact on the environment *outside* the site boundaries. (This is in contrast to health and safety, where the concern is for impact on people at their place of work. It is quite possible for something which has already been recognised as a health and safety issue to be an environmental issue as well, e.g. the effect of fire, discharges of fumes.) So, for a start, make a list of everything that leaves the site, through the gate, down the drains, and up the chimney stacks and exhaust vents.

Then turn your attention to what you buy. Where does it come from? What were the environmental impacts of making the products?

Next, what are the environmental aspects of your manufacturing processes or operations, in terms of resources, energy, waste and pollutant production? Everybody uses energy, in the form of electricity, gas, fuel oil, coal. This has consumed material resources, generating electricity has created carbon dioxide and other pollutants, burning gas does the same. Water is increasingly a scarce resource. Water down the drain is a waste and may carry pollutants.

As part of the review, make sure that you find, or draw up, a drainage plan for the site. Define all the drains and manholes. Where do the drains leave the site? Are they foul drains entering the water company's sewage system or are they land/storm water drains? Often these lead to streams or rivers. Is there a danger of pollution?

Do you use your own vehicles to make deliveries? Do you have a fleet of company cars? These use fuel and tyres (where disposal is a major environmental problem) and pollute the atmosphere.

How near are the nearest residential neighbours? Are they disturbed by your traffic, noise or smells?

Look at the site's housekeeping. Where are things stored? Can they leak? Is the ground protected or will it become contaminated? Is it generally tidy? A good standard of housekeeping not only impresses customers and your assessor in due course, but implies that people work in an orderly way; it also prevents waste through damage or deterioration.

Look at all your activities, not just manufacturing if you are a factory. Everybody needs to be committed to your environmental improvement programme. For example, the office will have computers (which use electricity and have a disposal problem), use paper (is it sourced from recycled paper or managed forests, do you segregate waste paper for recycling?), photocopiers and printers (where toners can be recycled). If you have a vending machine, what happens to the cups or empty cans? Toilets use electricity for lighting, sometimes all day and all night, and water, also sometimes all day and all night.

When you have made your list, compare it with the check list in Appendix B and see whether you have found everything. The field is so big that even the list in the appendix is not fully comprehensive but it covers most of the possibilities.

Measuring the environmental aspects

Now that the aspects are defined, you need to examine them further. Where does the aspect arise? How big is it? What and where is its impact?

For example, how many skips of general rubbish do you generate? What is in the rubbish? Where does it come from? Where does it go (presumably a landfill site somewhere)? What does it cost you each year?

How much electricity do you use, in units (kWh)? What does it cost you? Is this a real cost or an estimated usage? You need to know the real figures so you may need to take your own regular meter readings. Where is it used? Sub-metering can reveal a lot of useful information and can lead to substantial savings.

You can calculate how much carbon dioxide has been released as a result of the generation of this quantity of electricity. An example is given in the model Register of Environmental Aspects.

How much metallic scrap do you sell? Why does it arise? Asking the question often leads to ideas about how to improve the situation.

Work through each aspect and try to get a measure for each one.

Life cycle assessment

Life cycle assessment looks at the environmental impacts of a product from 'cradle to grave'. It therefore examines:

- The source of your raw materials and the physical resources, energy, pollution etc. involved in getting them to you.
- The resources etc. you use in creating your products from your raw materials and any pollution or waste you create in the process.
- What happens to your product in the long run e.g. will it be thrown away, can it be recycled, how long will it last, what energy, water etc. will it consume in its lifetime?

There is no written requirement in ISO 14001 to carry out life cycle assessments; they can be difficult to do and are certainly time-consuming. However, there is value in being aware of the principles of the subject as it will influence your evaluation of environmental aspects. It can also be particularly valuable when you come to designing new products or services. The concept has been incorporated in model Operating Procedure 14 'New products and processes'.

Compiling the Register of Environmental Aspects

The accompanying model Register of Environmental Aspects gives examples of aspects drawn from a range of organisations and shows how to describe an aspect. A blank form is included at the back of the Register.

Normal, abnormal and emergency situations

Note that the form contains a section that looks at the importance of an aspect in normal, abnormal and emergency situations. Not every aspect will necessarily exhibit all three characteristics, but some might and their importance needs to be recognised.

For example, a tank of diesel properly constructed, bunded and used will not cause any concern normally, but spillages might occur (abnormal) and a fire might be a disaster (emergency). A furnace process might give acceptable emissions when operating (normal) but give rise to black smoke when starting up (abnormal). Intermittent short duration use of noisy equipment could be classed as abnormal; so could minor gas leaks occurring when maintaining or reconfiguring plant and equipment. One company has registered the fact that toads when breeding cross an access road during one week of the year as an abnormal event.

This is one of the difficulties with environmental management systems. When you come to audit, a process is usually either working normally or is shut down. Yet most environmental disasters occur through abnormal or emergency conditions. Some of the biggest impacts have been caused by fire when drums of chemicals were not stored in a way that prevented the firemen's water washing the chemicals into a brook, or someone turned the wrong tap and let acid flood across the yard into the site drains. The importance of trying to predict what might happen cannot be stressed too much.

Significance of environmental aspects and legislation

You need some way of deciding which of the aspects are the most important and which therefore ought to be candidates for attention in the exercise of setting objectives and targets.

There are a number of ways of trying to work out relative significance. Some are very simple, some are very complicated. My experience as a consultant has led to me a scale which gives a significance range from 1 to 30, as shown in Fig. 6.1. By using a non-linear scale for severity, you will ensure that any event that causes a severe environmental impact, even if unlikely, will score highly enough on the impact scale to require management's attention.

When deciding on *severity*, you will need to make a judgement about how large an impact *your* activities make on the environment. For example, everybody knows that traffic is a major cause of atmospheric pollution. The temptation is therefore to give traffic a high severity rating; but if you have only two company cars, the impact will be far less than if you have a fleet of lorries and twenty salesmen on the road. So have regard to the scale of your activities that affect the environment.

Some aspects may have a high severity rating because of the risk of breaking the law. If by not paying sufficient attention to an aspect you risk prosecution, the harm to the organisation may not only be the cost of the fine but the damage to your reputation, both commercially and in the community.

Frequency of occurrence		Severity	
Description	Factor	Description	Factor
Unlikely (less than once a year)	1	Minimal environmental impact	1
Common (monthly/several times a year)	2	Low environmental impact	2
Frequent (daily/weekly)	3	Moderate environmental impact	3
		High environmental impact	6
		Severe environmental impact	10
Environmental Impact = Frequency of occurrence × Severity			

Fig. 6.1 Ranking the significance of environmental aspects

These rankings become more important when you come to decide on your environmental objectives and targets.

Reference to Operating Procedures

You will see that the form has a section titled Operating Procedures. In due course you will decide which of these aspects need to be managed in a formal way through writing and issuing Operating Procedures. These references will then be written in.

Cross referencing to regulations

There is also a section which cross refers to the Register of Environmental Legislation. Some of your aspects will be subject to regulation and it is useful to note this relationship. The converse will apply when you compile your Register of Environmental Legislation.

Legal and other requirements (Clause 4.3.2)

Defining the relevant legislation

In your policy you will be committing yourself to comply with all relevant environmental regulations and any other requirements such as an industry sector code of practice or the policy of a parent company. An example of one of the latter is the Responsible Care initiative of the Chemical Industries Association.

So how does an organisation set about finding out which of the raft of legislation applies to itself?

If you belong to a trade association or similar organisation, they probably have guidelines on relevant legislation for their industry sector (as published, for example, by the Engineering Employers Federation), and will issue guidelines as new legislation comes along. The association will also probably have a journal or newsletter which will have information about new regulations as they are issued. Your lawyers may have an environmental expert, but their time may be expensive. If you are using an environmental consultant you can expect him or her to know what is relevant. Otherwise, it is a good idea to subscribe to one of the reference books which are regularly updated, e.g. *Tolley's Environmental Law and Procedures Management*. This service is available for a cost which is usually less than £200 per year. The most common items of legislation are listed in Appendix C of this book, and these are outlined in the next section of the chapter.

The most frequent relevant legislation

The regulations applying to the following activities are those which most commonly apply:

- Wastes: Selection of waste carriers. Disposal of controlled wastes and special wastes. Special wastes are specifically defined, but are generally hazardous, toxic or dangerous substances. Controlled waste is everything else.
- Water: Effluents to foul sewer, surface drains.
- General nuisance: Noise, smoke, smells.
- Storage of flammable materials
- Contaminated land
- Planning consents: Planning consents may contain environmental conditions or restrictions, such as landscaping or limitations on car parking
- Packaging and packaging waste
- Prescribed processes: The *Environmental Protection (Prescribed Processes and Substances) Regulations 1991*, which are being replaced by the provisions of the *Pollution Prevention and Control Act 1999*, lists a large number of processes where the operator needs a licence from either the Environment Agency or the local authority.
- COSHH (*Control of Substances Hazardous to Health Regulations*): These specify maintenance requirements for local exhaust ventilation equipment.
- COMAH: Chemical processes may fall under the *Control of Major Hazard Regulations 1999*, which require risk assessments and emergency procedures that are acceptable to the Health and Safety Executive.

The Register of Environmental Legislation

The accompanying model Register of Environmental Legislation gives examples of how some of the regulations can be documented. A blank form is included at the back of the Register.

The question is always asked 'To what level of detail should I go when deciding which regulations to include in the Register?'

You will fairly easily compile a prime list of regulations which affect you directly. Then there are other regulations which impact on your business. For example, paying landfill tax is the responsibility of your waste carrier, but it certainly impacts indirectly on your costs; therefore it should be included, if only to remind your staff that every tonne sent to landfill costs you money. There will be other regulations which do not apply now, but which you need to be aware of for the possible future. For example, you may be below the threshold of the Packaging Regulations but if there is a chance that you will breach the threshold in a future year, include the regulations in your Register as a reminder.

Make sensible judgements. Do not include the *Bathing Water (Classification) Regulations* if your factory is inland and miles from the nearest beach.

Operating Procedures

This form also has a section titled Operating Procedures. You need to have a systematic way of ensuring that you comply with the legal requirements, and this is best done by writing Operating Procedures. Model Operating Procedures are included for some of the most common regulations.

Setting objectives and targets (Clause 4.3.3) (Step 5)

With your Registers complete and the significance of each item evaluated, management has the information it needs to set objectives.

The Standard gives the following guidance, saying that when setting objectives you should take into account:

- legal and other requirements;
- significant environmental aspects;
- technological options;
- financial, operational and business requirements;
- the views of interested parties.

Start by preparing a summary of the aspects in significance order. A blank form is included with model Operating Procedure 13, 'Environmental objectives and targets' and an example is given in Fig. 6.2.

Aspect	Impact (normal)	Impact (abnormal)	Impact (emergency)
Solvent usage and emissions	18	6	–
Raw materials	18	–	–
Fire	–	–	10
Electricity usage	9	–	–
Gas and gas oil usage	9	–	–
General rubbish	6	–	–
Paper usage	6	–	–
Packaging	6	–	–
Oven emissions (CO_2 etc.)	6	6	–
Transport	6	–	–
Water	3	–	–

Fig. 6.2 Environmental aspects – an example of a significance table

Table 6.1 Environmental objectives and targets

Solvents	Convert from 80% solvent-based/20% water based paints to 10% solvent based/90% water based in three years.
Raw materials – plastic granules	Reduce moulding rejections from 3% to 2%.
Electricity	Reduce usage by 10% over next 12 months.
Gas usage	Reduce usage by 10% over next 12 months.
Fire	Improve stocking arrangements for solvent drums and institute regular checks of sprinkler system.
General rubbish	Reduce number of skips sent out by 25% over next 12 months.
Packaging	Institute R&D programme to reduce quantity of packaging used by 20% within the next 12 months.
Oven emissions	Operator training in start-up and shut-down operations.

An objective is to make an improvement in an aspect in general. A target measures the amount of improvement you intend to achieve.

Objectives and targets which could be developed from the data in Fig. 6.2 are shown in Table 6.1.

This is the time to give thought to good technical operation. A number of acronyms are in use which you will come across in the technical literature, including:

- BPEO: best practicable environmental option;
- BAT: best available techniques.

If you already hold a licence under the Environment Protection Act Part 1, you may well have a condition imposed to achieve best technical performance within a given timescale. Even if it is not being forced on you, be aware that there are specifications for good performance, e.g. emissions of particulates from chimneys ought not to exceed $50\,mg$ per m^3.

It is a good idea to develop a range of improvement objectives such that as many people in the organisation as possible are involved. This should extend to include administrative staff as much as production and technical staff. In this way the environmental culture will gradually spread throughout the whole organisation. Recycling programmes and energy saving are obvious examples.

If you want help on how to improve environmental performance, there is a lot of useful information readily available about good practice. In particular, the Environment Agency and the Department for Environment, Food and Rural Affairs (DEFRA) have many publications dealing with pollution, water and energy, many of which are free. A description of the types of information available and contact addresses etc. are given in Appendix D.

Environmental management programme (Clause 4.3.4)

The objectives and targets now have to be turned into an action plan. The essential decisions are:

- Who should be in charge?
- Who else will be involved?
- What sequence of steps/actions will lead to the end result?
- What is the timetable?

Your assessor will expect you to show positive control of the process. A suitable form for setting out and progressing the plan is included with model Operating Procedure 13 'Environmental objectives and targets'. You will also need Operating Procedures to keep control of your important aspects, your statutory responsibilities and to control your EMS. The process of defining and writing procedures is described in Chapter 7.

Chapter 7

Implementation and operation

Introduction

ISO 14001 Clause 4.4 is concerned with the implementation of the environmental management system and its operation.

The clause requires that:

- You have defined the organisation and people's responsibilities and have provided sufficient resources to do the job properly.
- The people involved have been trained and are competent, and are aware of the environmental implications of their jobs.
- You have a system for handling internal and external communications.
- Documents are properly controlled.
- The operational activities are properly controlled. This probably calls for writing Operating Procedures.
- The procedures extend to the involvement of suppliers and subcontractors.
- You are prepared for any emergencies.

Each of these will be considered in turn.

Structure and responsibility (ISO 14001 Clause 4.4.1)

Organisation

This is where you need an organisation chart on which appears each person, described by job title, who has any part to play in the EMS. This will range from the managing director or chief executive at the top down to the key operatives at the bottom. The chart will be included in your Environmental Manual.

You will also need to include with the chart a mini-job description for the key players and a general statement about the environmental responsibilities of other people. If you are a large organisation, this amount of detail could overload your manual. In this case, put in a chart showing the main organisational features, and refer the reader to detailed departmental charts and job descriptions, which would probably be held by a personnel department. Then you need to check that the job descriptions do in fact contain the references to environmental responsibilities.

Resources

Management is charged with the responsibility for providing the necessary resources to implement the EMS, in people and the relevant skills, technology, finance etc. The best way to deal with this is to make it an agenda item at your management review meetings.

Environmental manager

The Standard then calls for the appointment of the 'management representative(s)'. The appointment of an environmental manager who will drive the project was discussed in Chapter 5. This person is responsible for:

- ensuring the creation and implementation of the EMS;
- monitoring performance and reporting to top management.

These duties will be written into the Environmental Management Manual.

Training, awareness and competence (Clause 4.4.2)

As in a quality system, there is a need to identify training needs for all the people involved in the EMS. The training must then be given and records kept. If you have a training procedure in existence in the quality system, it can be enlarged to include environment. Model Operating Procedure 15 'Environmental training' shows how this can be done.

The Standard is quite specific about what employees need to know. In short, these are:

- the importance of conforming to the policy and procedures of the EMS;
- knowing the significant environmental aspects of their job;
- roles and responsibilities in relation to the EMS;
- the potential consequences of departing from the Operating Procedures.

The organisation has to demonstrate that employees, and particularly those who have a key environmental role, are competent to carry out their responsibilities. This can be on the basis of education, experience and/or training.

So it is essential that people really do understand the importance of their job. One way of doing this is to write the environmental features, risks and safety actions into specific Operating Procedures or Work Instructions. Model Operating Procedures 5 'Furnace operations' and 6 'Water treatment plant' are examples.

Author's note: ISO 9004: 2000, the guidelines for implementing ISO 9001: 2000, also now suggests that people should be trained to be aware of the consequences of not doing their job properly.

Communication (Clause 4.4.3)

The organisation is required to have a formal procedure for:

- passing environmental information etc. between people within the organisation;
- handling communications with people from outside the organisation, not forgetting the regulators, such as the Environment Agency.

You also have to take a decision whether or not to publicise information about your aspects or simply to respond to questions when asked.

These are best dealt with by writing an Operating Procedure; model Operating Procedure 16 'Environmental communications' is an example.

Environmental management system documentation (Clause 4.4.4)

The Standard requires that the 'core elements of the management system and their interaction' shall be described, and that the related documentation shall be sign-posted. The description can either be in paper or electronic form, thus recognising that paperless systems are becoming more and more common.

The easiest and most usual way of meeting this requirement is to write an Environmental Management Manual which will link together the clauses of the Standard, your Registers, Operating Procedures, and the various forms and documents used to manage and report on your environmental system. Any licence issued by the Environment Agency or local authority is an essential part of the documented system.

Chapter 9 gives detailed guidance on how to write the manual.

Document control (Clause 4.4.5)

Anyone who has a quality management system will be familiar with the practice of document control.

Briefly, documents which run the EMS including the manual, the Registers, the Operating Procedures and any Work Instructions must be 'controlled', i.e. be authorised, be distributed to the right people who will receive revisions automatically, be regularly reviewed to ensure that they stay relevant to changing practices and obsolete documents will be removed from circulation.

Document control also extends to any necessary reference documents. Chapter 6 has referred to the need to keep up to date with relevant legislation. How you do this will be written into your document control procedure. ISO 14001 itself is a reference document that will be revised in due course.

Model Operating Procedure 17 'Document control' describes a way of meeting these requirements. If you already have a similar procedure in your quality management system, you will be able to adapt it by adding the titles of the environmental documents to your existing quality titles.

The clause also makes reference to documents being legible, dated, readily identifiable, decently filed and with specified retention times. This latter point is reiterated in more detail in Chapter 8 under 'Records' and is better dealt with there.

Operational control (Clause 4.4.6) (Step 6)

Introduction

This is the key part of this clause. The Registers create the foundation of the EMS; the procedures are its heart. Operating Procedures drive the EMS. They are not only needed to control processes but also to manage the EMS itself.

Although this part of the Standard is only concerned with processes, it is convenient to deal with the total need for Operating Procedures at this stage, e.g.:

- processes
- emergencies
- administration.

Control of processes

Chapter 6 noted that procedures will be needed to control the key environmental aspects and to ensure compliance with relevant legislation. You may also require procedures to progress your improvement plans, or these may evolve as you progress through the stages of the action plan.

Remember that you will have identified certain processes as being linked to an environmental aspect. Control of these processes will require an Operating Procedure, but it is highly likely that you already have an Operating Procedure or Work Instruction for managing the process itself. In this case, write the environmental dimension into your existing text. The procedure now becomes a part of your EMS as well as being part of your quality management system. The same applies to maintenance.

Possible titles for Operating Procedures linked to processes are:

- Waste handling and segregation.
- Disposal of controlled wastes.
- Disposal of special waste.
- Compliance with conditions imposed by any operating licence.
- Control of effluents, drainage.
- Compliance with 'Packaging Waste' Regulations.
- Control of the environmental aspects of particular processes (which is best written into existing procedures or Work Instructions if possible).
- Storage facilities.
- Housekeeping, to prevent pollution, land contamination, etc.
- Energy control and monitoring.

- Laboratories.
- Fuel economy, e.g. selection of vehicles, good driving practice.
- Control of environmental aspects of goods and services from suppliers and subcontractors (which may be written into site or contract instructions).
- Taking environmental considerations into account when planning new developments.

Links to health and safety

There are other existing management controls, particularly health and safety, which need to be linked to and cross-referenced in your EMS. For example, if you have local exhaust ventilation equipment (LEVs), they exhaust to atmosphere and so can have an environmental impact. It is likely that their maintenance requirement under the COSHH Regulations (not less than every 14 months) will be included in your Health and Safety Policy or in your planned maintenance system. If you transport dangerous goods, you will almost certainly have existing procedures or instructions governing these.

Emergencies

The next sub clause of the Standard deals with emergencies, and will be discussed later in this chapter. For the moment, we need to take note that emergency procedures need to be part of the EMS, or if part of another system, e.g. health and safety, or free-standing, e.g. COSHH, they will need to be cross-referred, e.g.:

- Fire.
- Control of dangerous or polluting spillages.
- COMAH emergency plans (if relevant).

Administration of the EMS

The need for some administrative Operating Procedures has already been noted e.g. communications, document control. Others will be required by later clauses of the Standard. These are shown in the box below, which also notes which of them coincide with procedures that will already be in your ISO 9001 quality management system. These can be made dual purpose by adding the appropriate words. Refer to model Operating Procedures 15 and 17–21.

- Control of Registers.
- Setting and progressing environmental objectives and targets.
- Training (consolidate with ISO 9001).
- Communications.
- Document control (consolidate with ISO 9001).
- Suppliers and subcontractors (consolidate with ISO 9001).
- Control of measuring and process control equipment (consolidate with ISO 9001).
- Nonconformance, corrective and preventive action, including external complaints (consolidate with ISO 9001).
- Environmental records (consolidate with ISO 9001).
- Internal audits (consolidate with ISO 9001).
- Management review.

Writing Operating Procedures

When writing a procedure, be aware of the different gradations of meaning, as shown in the following list:

- shall – do it every time
- will – do it every time
- may – this means optional (be careful not to allow too much freedom)
- should – ought to do it every time, but not mandatory – (another word to avoid)
- could – this means optional
- instructions – to be followed in every detail
- guidelines – to be used as guides, typically for trained staff, and can be adapted if necessary.

The Standard also requires that you state the operating criteria in procedures. This is not always possible, but operational limits should be set if possible.

If consent limits have been imposed and you have a system of regular or continuous monitoring, remember to set your trigger levels tighter than the consent levels. Then if an alarm sounds you have time to catch the situation *before* the consent level is breached.

When you set about writing procedures it is essential that you involve the people who are already doing the job. They are the experts. They know what happens and where things can go wrong. Often they have written aide-memoires to themselves to remind themselves what to do in certain circumstances; these are ideal raw material for the formal procedures you are going to write. Not only will these people be a great help to you, but the fact that they have been involved at the outset (and you will of course refer back to them as the work progresses) means that they will have a sense of ownership when the EMS is launched.

Emergency preparedness and response (Clause 4.4.7)

The type of procedures which may be required are noted above, whether they are an actual part of the EMS or cross-referenced to it.

When writing these procedures, remember to include that:

- procedures should be periodically tested if possible, e.g. fire drills or a mock situation;
- if you have a real emergency, you should hold a post-mortem to check how well the procedures worked, and revise them if necessary in the light of experience.

Emergency procedures should be written as a list of short, sharp statements that can be clearly understood. You can even use a larger and bolder type face than usual. If they are ever required, the reader will not have time to digest complicated sentences when everybody around them is trying not to panic.

Work Instructions

So far we have assumed that Operating Procedures alone are adequate to control the organisation's activities. In small organisations this may well be the case, but in larger organisations it may be desirable to introduce another level of documentation, the 'Work Instruction', which states how a particular job is to be carried out in detail. This prevents the Operating Procedures becoming overloaded with detail, and can aid the process of keeping documentation up-to-date; it is easier to change and re-issue a one-page Work Instruction than a multi-page procedure.

Examples of more detailed Work Instructions could be:

- How to carry out the analysis of an effluent in the laboratory.
- How to collect the data and carry out calculations necessary to fill in the 'packaging waste' return to the Environment Agency.

Even in small organisations there may be a case for Work Instructions. For example, model Operating Procedure 3 'Waste handling and segregation' describes how wastes might be segregated. This could be backed up by notices on the walls at each place where waste is created reminding people what to do with it. These notices would be controlled as Work Instructions.

If you only have a few Work Instructions, rather than create a new layer of documentation, it may be easier to include them as appendices to the associated Operating Procedures.

Another aspect relating to Work Instructions is this. A Work Instruction *tells* people how to do a job. Training *teaches* people how to do a job. If the training is comprehensive and the training record shows that the training has been given, it may not be necessary to write the Work Instruction at all.

Chapter 8

Checking, corrective action and management review

Monitoring and measurement (Clause 4.5.1)

Introduction

This clause of the Standard has three parts:

- Measuring impacts to monitor performance and to track progress towards the objectives and targets.
- Calibration and maintenance of measuring equipment.
- Evaluating compliance with the relevant environmental legislation and regulations.

Measuring performance

Chapter 6 dealt with defining the starting position, defining and measuring the environmental aspects. Quantities of rubbish generated, units of electricity consumed and weight of scrap generated were given as three examples. For each objective or target, you need a means of being able to say whether you are winning or not.

Although the principle of measurement is included here, the practice is best carried out at the objective setting stage, and has therefore been included in Procedure 13 'Environmental objectives and targets'.

Calibration and measuring equipment

As in ISO 9001, monitoring and measuring equipment must be calibrated and maintained and records kept so that there is evidence that the equipment is sufficiently accurate for its purpose.

You may have measuring equipment built into your processes to keep them under control, or you may take measurements in order to plot your progress towards objectives. Do remember that your measuring equipment only needs to be sufficiently accurate for the purpose. If all you want is to show a trend, the degree of accuracy required will be less than if you have to keep operating parameters within a tight range, or you have safety systems which trigger alarms or shut-down routines if a process is going out of control.

Again you may find that equipment needed for environmental purposes is already listed and calibrated as part of a quality management system.

Examples of equipment could be:

- weighbridges;
- thermocouples (for example, if you are a drum reconditioner, best practice requires that the vapours released in the oven are heated to at least 850°C for at least 2 seconds to burn off the chemicals safely);
- VOC sampling equipment (for example, if under the terms of an operating licence you have to monitor the concentration of VOCs emitted from a stack);
- laboratory equipment (for example, if you have to analyse samples of effluent);
- meters, for measuring electricity, gas or water consumptions.

Model Operating Procedure 18 'Monitoring and measuring equipment' describes a way of meeting the requirements. If you already have a similar procedure in your quality management system, you will be able to adapt it by adding the extra equipment to the list of equipment requiring calibration.

Compliance with environmental legislation and regulations

The Standard requires that the organisation periodically evaluates compliance with the relevant environmental legislation and regulations. The easiest way to do this is to follow the suggestion in Chapter 7 that you write Operating Procedures to describe how you ensure you observe the relevant legislation. Then your internal audit schedule will routinely check that they are being followed in practice.

Nonconformance and corrective and preventive action (Clause 4.5.2)

Introduction

'Nonconformance' is officially defined as 'The non-fulfilment of the specified requirement'. It is better defined as 'Something which has happened which is not in accordance with the planned way of doing things'.

Many people find the word 'nonconformance' is off-putting. Despite the principle underlying both ISO 14001 and ISO 9001 that we learn from our mistakes and take steps to prevent them happening again and by doing so gradually improve performance, the very sound of the word has a negative connotation and can lead people to viewing the whole management system in the same way. For this reason, some organisations abandon the word and use 'incident' or 'problem' instead.

Because it is the official terminology, we shall continue to use the word 'nonconformance' here, but think hard about which word is the best to use in your organisation. If 'Incident Report' or 'Problem Report' will make life easier, then use it. The model form in Operating Procedure 19 'Nonconformance, corrective and preventive action' has been titled 'Nonconformance/Incident Report' in an attempt to satisfy both schools of thought.

Causes of nonconformance

Deviations from what is intended can arise in a number of ways, including:

- failure to follow an Operating Procedure;
- the procedure is inadequate;
- an equipment failure;
- an unforeseen emergency for which no emergency plan has been prepared.

If these lead to an environmental incident such as the release of a quantity of prohibited material into the atmosphere or into the effluent or drains, there must obviously be a procedure for correcting or mitigating the situation in the short term and examining whether a procedural change or a new procedure is needed to prevent a repetition.

The internal auditing programme should throw up any instances of procedures not being followed which, even if they have not caused an incident so far, might yet do so. These findings therefore have to be acted upon.

Lastly, any environmental complaint from outside the organisation, which might be from a statutory body like the Environment Agency or a water company or from a member of the general public, will require investigation and possible corrective and preventive action. These last will of course have been recognised through the Operating Procedure on 'Communication', but here is the best place to say what to do about them.

Operating Procedure for nonconformities

In a quality management system, the word 'nonconformity' is most usually applied to nonconforming product and the procedure revolves around isolating the offending articles and deciding what to do with them. The reporting system is designed to handle this type of situation.

In an environmental management system, the nonconformity will be associated with actions, events or situations. A different style of reporting will probably be required, and the nature of immediate corrective action, investigation and deciding whether longer term preventive action is required and what that action should be will also be different.

It is also quite likely that prevention will require a change in a procedure, an outcome that is recognised in the Standard, and one that must be recorded.

In these circumstances it is probably better to write a new environmental Operating Procedure than try to adapt an existing quality procedure. Model Operating Procedure 19 'Nonconformance, corrective and preventive action' shows one way of doing this.

The procedure is required to address the following issues:

- Responsibility and authority for handling and investigating the nonconformity.
- Action to deal with any impacts caused.
- Taking corrective and preventive action.
- The action must be appropriate to the size of the problem and the environmental impact.
- Records must be kept.

Records (Clause 4.5.3)

The Standard requires you to have a procedure for identifying and looking after your environmental records. The simplest way to define an 'environmental record' is to treat any document used in carrying out any procedure as being part of the environmental management system.

Some of the documents will have legal status, such as Controlled Waste Transfer Notes, and these have a designated retention time. If you have an operating licence, the terms of the licence may say how long records should be kept. You are strongly recommended to have a central repository for legal documents. This can be with the environmental manager, or in accounts or with the company secretary etc.

Other documents record your physical environmental performance. You can decide how long these need to be kept.

Documents which record the performance and progress of the management system itself such as notes of management meetings and audit reports should be kept for three years. Your assessor is probably going to be required to carry out an overall review of your performance every three years and may need to refer back to earlier events.

The Standard requires records to be legible. This can be quite a challenge for some people, and makes sense of the arrangement on many documents, especially legal ones, that the person signing it also prints his or her name. Make sure this happens.

Documents must be identifiable. Use the test that if someone spilt the contents of the filing cabinet on the floor, could you put everything back in the right place?

Documents must also be protected against damage. Faxes on thermal paper can fade, so make a rule that such faxed records are photocopied before being filed.

The Standard says records must be retrievable. It does not say they must be retrievable instantly so there is nothing to stop you archiving them, provided you can demonstrate that you know where they are and that they can be accessed if needed.

Model Operating Procedure 20 'Environmental records' addresses these issues.

Environmental management system audit (Clause 4.5.4)

This is one of the most important, and certainly one of the most powerful ways of maintaining control of an organisation and, if used to its full potential, to improve the organisation's performance.

Model Operating Procedure 21 'Internal environmental audits' sets out how to observe the requirements of the Standard. Because of the key role that auditing should play in the organisation's management, the whole of Chapter 11 has been devoted to this subject.

Management review (Clause 4.6)

No organisation can be allowed to operate and develop without the top management regularly keeping an eye on things. How this is done will vary from daily 'morning meetings' dealing with immediate problems to board meetings that take the long view.

All management standards, and ISO 14001 is no exception, require periodic reviews of performance to ensure, in the words of the Standard, 'continuing stability, adequacy and effectiveness'. You need to establish how frequently meetings will be held and at what level in the organisation.

We have already come across a top management activity in the setting of environmental objectives and targets and establishing the management programme. It makes sense to combine the above planning activities with the review activities in one meeting. Model Operating Procedure 22 'Management review' describes how this can be done.

Chapter 9

The Environmental Management Manual (Step 7)

Introduction

All the building blocks of the EMS are now in place, the Registers and Operating Procedures (backed up by any Work Instructions and forms) are written. Now you have to put the roof on top of the structure to bind it all together by writing an Environmental Management Manual.

Many people think they have to write their manual at the start of the project. Such manuals can tend to be full of pious words of good intentions and parrot phrases from the Standard. Then it has to be re-written once the EMS has become a reality to bring it up-to-date. It is far better to leave writing the manual until the rest of the work has been done.

The purpose of the manual

The manual serves a number of purposes:

- It links the component parts of your EMS to the clauses and requirements of the Standard.
- The act of writing it helps you to check that you have addressed all the clauses and requirements of the Standard.
- It gives your assessor a guide to the structure of your EMS, so that he/she knows where to look to find how each clause of the Standard is satisfied.
- Lastly, if a customer asks you to prove that you as a management are in control of your environmental responsibilities, you can let them have a copy of the manual.

Arising from this last point, you need to be careful that you do not include any confidential information in the manual. Anything confidential should be kept in the Operating Procedures. The Operating Procedures say how you actually run the organisation. They are yours, for the use of your staff only.

Planning the manual

A tip: when writing the manual, have your copy of ISO 14001 open in front of you. Look at each sentence or clause in the Standard in turn. Then write down where in your EMS you deal with that subject. Check that you have dealt with all the requirements of the clause. If you find something missing, fill in the gap before going any further.

Manuals and operating procedures are different types of document

When you wrote your Operating Procedures, you used the words 'shall' or 'will'. Procedures are *instructions*. The manual *describes* your EMS. The wording therefore is 'the organisation/ company/business *does* something', i.e. it is written in the present tense.

It is because of this difference in emphasis and the different purposes served by the manual and the Operating Procedures that you are strongly advised to keep them as two separate documents. Do not be tempted to combine them.

Another good reason for keeping them separate is that you will almost certainly be changing one or other of the Operating Procedures quite often, whereas, with luck, the manual will be a more stable document. You do not want to have to re-issue your manual just because of a change in a working practice.

Contents of a manual

Structure

A model Environmental Management Manual is included as part of this book. It has the following structure:

- The Environmental Policy
- Issue and amendment control sheet
- Contents
- Introduction to the organisation
- A summary of what is contained in the Registers and Operating Procedures, laid out so that the text corresponds to each clause of ISO 14001.

The numbering system

You will notice that the introductory pages are numbered 0, so that when the reader comes to the body of the document it is possible for the paragraph numbering to be aligned with the numbering of the clauses in the Standard.

The introduction

The introduction introduces your organisation to the reader. Describe what you do, e.g. manufacturer of plastic cases, transport fleet operator, solicitor. If it would be helpful, mention your main processes and your main types of customers.

Give an indication of how big you are either in number of employees or the area of your site, and say where you are located geographically.

If you are regulated by the Environment Agency or your local authority, say who is the regulator and which of the processes listed in the Environmental Protection (Prescribed Processes and Substances) Regulations 1991 or the Pollution Prevention and Control Act 1999 apply to you. Also say if you are a COMAH site.

If you are already registered to ISO 9001, state this at the end.

The clauses of the standard

Now you come to the purpose of the manual: to show how you meet the requirements of the Standard. The manual also acts as a sign-posting document to all the building blocks, i.e. the Registers and the Operating Procedures.

So each clause or sub-clause of the manual first states how the requirements of the corresponding clause of the Standard have been satisfied, and then lists the related Operating Procedures.

Author's note: if you are a large organisation with a lot of Operating Procedures, this arrangement can make the manual look very disjointed. You may be better advised to list all the clauses and sub-clauses and the related Operating Procedures as a table in an appendix, and refer to this in section 1 of the manual. This alternative has been included as an 'OR' paragraph. Such an Appendix A is included in the model Environmental Management Manual.

You need to list *all* the clauses and sub-clauses of the Standard. If any of them do not apply, you need to say so.

References to the quality management system

If you have drawn on any of your existing quality system Operating Procedures by adding environmental wording or references to them, then these will be quoted as though they are Environmental Operating Procedures in their own right. This possibility is also included in the appropriate places as an 'OR' paragraph.

Organisation charts

Clause 4.4.1 refers to your management organisation and ideally requires an organisation chart. The level of detail you show depends on the complexity and size of your management structure; this has already been discussed in Chapter 7. You need to decide whether you will include the chart within the text of your manual at clause 4.4.1, or whether it will be more convenient to include it as an appendix.

As it is likely that your 'environmental manager' will be carrying out these duties in addition to his/her existing job, do not forget to identify who the environmental manager is on the chart.

Chapter 10
The launch (Step 8)

Introduction

Up to now, we have been dealing with the *creation* of the Environmental Management System (EMS). This is all preparation for putting the EMS into *action*.

Although Chapter 5 recommended that Operating Procedures (and any related Work Instructions) should be given to the relevant people as soon as they have been drafted so that they can see how well they work in practice and to what extent they really match current practice, there comes a time when it is desirable to say to everybody 'The environmental system is complete. We now have to check it out and get ready for our assessment'.

The decision to adopt a formal EMS has already affected, or will soon affect, the majority of people in the organisation. They were all involved at the 'commitment' stage. Now they need to be brought up to date. It is well worthwhile planning a systematic launching programme which will include another communication session or sessions.

Chapter 5 listed the component parts of the launch as:

- The first formal environmental management review meeting.
- Planning document distribution.
- The communication session.
- Organising any extra training required.

Management meeting

Whilst Operating Procedure 22 contains the standard agenda for environmental management review meetings, this comes into play once the EMS is in operation. At this stage, you only need the following agenda items:

- Approval or adoption of the documented EMS.
- Agree the plans for the communication exercise which will launch the programme.
- Decide on any specific training needs.
- Agree the forward timetable leading to assessment.

The documented EMS needs to be formally adopted by the board or the top management team for two reasons:

- It ensures top level commitment to the project.
- It sets the date when the EMS came into being. This is a marker for the assessor, since he or she cannot hold you responsible, and so cannot find noncompliances, for any failures to follow the requirements of the EMS that occurred prior to this date.

Make sure the meeting is minuted.

Planning document distribution

Introduction

It is all too easy to say that every person who plays a part in the EMS should have their own copy of the documentation. Unfortunately, this floods the place with paper, itself undesirable from an environmental viewpoint, and it turns the environmental manager's job of controlling the documents and keeping them up-to-date into a nightmare.

So before you start on the public launch of the EMS, think hard about how you are going to distribute your documents, particularly the Operating Procedures and any Work Instructions.

The manual and Registers

Often you can manage with just one copy of the Environmental Management Manual and the Registers. If your Operating Procedures are sufficiently comprehensive they will contain all the information needed for the day-to-day running of the organisation. So a master copy of the manual and the Registers held by the Environmental Manager may suffice, so long as everybody who might need to refer to them knows where they are kept. This means they should be visible, not hidden in a drawer or bookcase.

The policy

The one exception to the above is the Environmental Policy. Include a copy of this with each copy of the Operating Procedures, and post it on the key notice boards and in reception.

The Operating Procedures

Obviously each Operating Procedure needs to be readily available to all the *relevant* people, right down to the shop or office floor. An effective way of doing this is to decide which sections of the site need all or some of the procedures, e.g. workshop, security, general office. Place the relevant procedures in a brightly coloured ring binder – choose a colour not used for any other purpose – and put it into a wall mounted holder in an obvious place, e.g. by the notice board or near the entrance to a mess room.

Make one person such as the local supervisor the official 'holder' of the ring binder.

The Work Instructions

Work Instructions need to be displayed at the place where the particular job they refer to is carried out.

Communication

As explained earlier, you will have been implementing your procedures as you go along, but now is the time to carry out your next communication exercise. Bring people together to give them:

- A brief description of the work done in the initial review and the compilation of the Register of Environmental Aspects and the Register of Environmental Legislation. Liven the discussion by comparing your thoughts with theirs about what is most relevant to the organisation.
- Set out the environmental improvement objectives for Year One.
- Describe the Operating Procedures, what they cover, how they have been distributed, where they have been located. In particular mention those that are especially relevant to the members of the particular audience.
- Tell the audience to read their procedures and invite them to feed back comments and suggestions. If no comments are forthcoming, it will become a job for auditors in due course to obtain feedback.
- Explain that the whole EMS will now be checked by internal auditors. Announce the names of the auditors. Make it quite clear that the auditors are on *your* and *their* side, and are part of the process of making sure the EMS is right as well as checking that it is working properly.

- Set out the timetable for internal auditing and assessment.
- Explain that there will be another communication session just before the assessment takes place.

Organise this communication in the same way as your organised the first communication sessions described in Chapter 5. If you are briefing managers or supervisors who will then pass the message on, give them a briefing note so that the message is everywhere consistent.

Training

Chapter 7 described the requirements set out in Clause 4.4.2 of the Standard for training and this is amplified in model Operating Procedure 15.

Because of the number of people involved and the need for them all to know what their particular responsibilities and duties are, an early start on the training programme is essential if you do not want a panic as the date of the assessment approaches.

This is not as forbidding a task as it might seem. Remember that most people are doing their job adequately already; all that you have done is codify what they do into formal procedures. Nevertheless, in carrying out your review at the start of the project you probably came across some necessary activities which were not being done at all or not being done consistently.

The first requirement is that everybody should be aware of the organisation's commitment to the environment (the Environmental Policy) and the fact that there is an Environmental Management System in operation. They need to know where 'their' copy of the Operating Procedures is located, and they need to be alert to any particular environmental responsibilities which affect them. All these points can be covered in the launch communication. Keep a record of the names of everybody who attends and enter the event on their training record under the heading 'Environmental and ISO14001 awareness'.

We are into personal training when it comes to making sure that each individual knows the significant environmental aspects of their job and the potential consequences of departing from the Operating Procedures. It may be sufficient for supervisors to take each person in their teams through the relevant procedures. On the other hand it can be a job for the training department if you have one. However it is organised, make sure the relevant entries get onto the training record.

The last thing you want to happen at the assessment is for the assessor to say to an individual 'Have you been trained in the environmental implications of your job'? and for the answer to be 'No'. My experience is that this happens all too frequently, even when the people are competent but somehow are unaware that they have been trained.

Chapter 11
Internal environmental auditing (Step 9)

Introduction

Clause 4.5.4 of the Standard requires the organisation to have an auditing programme and auditing procedures to determine that the Environmental Management System (EMS) is working as planned, and to ensure that there shall be feedback of the results to management. Anyone who has experience of a quality management system will be accustomed to this activity.

As stated in Chapter 8, the internal auditing process is an extremely powerful tool for maintaining and improving an organisation's performance. Unfortunately, many people regard it as a chore, because it takes the auditors away from their regular jobs which are already time consuming; the people being audited likewise can resent the interruption to their work. Some people also are not happy about being 'checked up on' by outsiders.

Auditing *must* be carried out, and it is up to the management to provide the necessary resources and give the process their full support. This can be done as part of the launch process described in Chapter 10.

This chapter is not about how to carry out audits, this is dealt with in the training your auditors will receive, but it discusses some of the organisational aspects of auditing which are included in model Operating Procedure 21. These are:

- The audit programme (or schedule).
- Selection and training of auditors.
- Reporting the findings.

The audit programme

The first question is 'How often should each part of the EMS be audited?' The Standard gives guidance to the extent of saying 'periodic' audits and that the programme 'shall be based on the environmental importance of the activity concerned and the results of previous audits'.

For an EMS that has been assessed, most assessors will accept that auditing everything once a year is adequate, unless the activity is particularly important or the last audit threw up problems which make it desirable to organise a repeat audit soon afterwards to check that what was wrong or incomplete has been corrected.

However, in the time between launching your EMS and the assessment you must audit the *whole* system, and any troublesome areas will need to be reaudited. The value of audits in this stage of the implementation of the EMS is threefold:

- They give the people being audited an opportunity to discuss the Operating Procedures, which throws up any errors in the procedures themselves or can lead to suggestions which will improve the procedures.
- They reveal any places where the implementation of a procedure has not been completed, and initiates a corrective action with a completion date.
- Lastly, where the Operating Procedures have been implemented, an audit shows whether they are being followed.

In order to ensure that the audit programme comprehensively checks the whole EMS, it can be helpful to draw up a schedule which groups the procedures under the relevant clause of the Standard, and then to compile a programme which includes all the clauses. This system has been used in the model Operating Procedure 21. Figure 11.1 shows what the allocation

Topic	ISO 14001 Clause	Manual Ref.	Related documents
Environmental management system	4.1	1	–
Environmental policy	4.2	2	–
Environmental aspects	4.3.1	3.1	Register of Environmental Aspects; OP 13 Section 3; OP 21 Section 3
Legal requirements	4.3.2	3.2	Register of Environmental Legislation; OP 17 Section 5.3
Objectives, targets, management programme	4.3.3, 4.3.4	3.3, 3.4	OP 13 Section 4
Structure and responsibility	4.4.1	4.1	–
Training, awareness and competence	4.4.2	4.2	OP 15
Communication	4.4.3	4.3	OP 16
Documentation, document control	4.4.4, 4.4.5	4.4, 4.5	OP 17
Operational control	4.4.6	4.6	
Waste handling and disposal			OP 1, OP 2, OP 3
Solvents			OP 4
Furnace			OP 5
Water treatment plant			OP 6
Packaging			OP 7
etc.			
Emergencies	4.4.7	4.7	
Fire			Action in case of fire
etc.			
Monitoring and measurement	4.5.1	5.1	OP 13 Section 5
Nonconformance, corrective & preventive action	4.5.2	5.2	OP 19
Records	4.5.3	5.3	OP 20
EMS audits	4.5.4	5.4	OP 21
Management review	4.6	6	OP 22

Fig. 11.1 Audit topics

schedule might look like. If there are too many procedures associated with one clause for them to be audited on one occasion, then divide them up into sub-groups. This can particularly apply to Clause 4.4.6 'Operational control'.

Many people allocate audit topics to particular months of the year. Most people have experience of circumstances which make it difficult to keep precisely to the programme, yet if you fail to keep to the programme you are in danger of collecting a minor non-compliance from your assessor. Give yourself some leeway; a way of doing this has been included in the text of model Operating Procedure 21.

Selecting and training of auditors

Selection of auditors

Who will you choose to be your environmental auditors? If you are registered to ISO 9001, you will already have people who have been trained in the art of auditing. Would they be suitable as environmental auditors as well?

The structure of an EMS can be divided into two parts:

- The administration of the EMS, which is almost an exact parallel to the administration of ISO 9001.
- The Operating Procedures that control environmental activities and aspects throughout the organisation.

Quality auditors should have no difficulty in auditing the administrative activities.

When it comes to auditing environmental activities, it is important that the auditors should understand the processes and the implications of the processes that they are auditing, whilst still being managerially independent of the process itself.

Auditing only has real purpose when there is a dialogue between the auditor and the people being audited about what is going on, rather than a sterile question and answer session. In this way can you be sure that the audit has been properly comprehensive and that the auditor has been able to pick up and recognise the implications of any changes to plant, processes or systems that could have an impact on the organisation's environmental performance, and therefore need to be incorporated into the EMS.

There is another option, which is to use an outside registered environmental auditor. If you have used consultants (see Chapter 5) they may offer a service at a reasonable cost. The service may also include maintaining your EMS documentation for you. If you choose this path you will have confidence that environmental developments are being correctly evaluated and followed up.

Training

So, having chosen your auditors, how should they be trained?

The Standard makes no reference to training auditors other than saying under the 'Training' clause that people must have received appropriate training in order to be able to exercise their environmental responsibilities. ISO 14004 says that auditors must be 'properly trained' without any guidance as to what this means.

One thing is certain. Your assessor will want to know what training your auditors have had.

Remember that you are not expecting your auditors to audit your EMS against the Standard. This will have been done by your assessor at the time of assessment. You require that your auditors tell you whether:

- the Operating Procedures are being observed in practice or not;
- things have changed so that an Operating Procedure needs updating;
- there have been any developments which should be incorporated into the EMS;
- anything has happened which compromises observance of the Standard.

So you are looking for basic or foundation training, not lead or advanced training.

Unlike ISO 9001, ISO 14001 contains the requirement to define the relevant environmental legislation and abide by it and to determine environmental aspects. This means that the internal environmental auditors need to be more aware of what is going on *outside* the boundaries of the organisation than is the case with quality auditors at present. A similar requirement to observe the regulatory and legal obligations relating to the product or service being provided is now included in ISO 9001: 2000.

Ways of training internal auditors, in an order of preference, are:

- Courses run by the assessing bodies themselves. Some of these run a one-day conversion course for quality auditors.
- Courses run by consulting firms or colleges that have been approved by IEMA.
- Courses which are run by a registered environmental auditor, probably from a local consultancy firm.
- Sending one member of staff on one of the above courses, and then using him/her to train others, by auditing alongside them until they are deemed to be skilled enough to work alone.

One effective way of training if you are prepared to pay for it is to invite a local registered auditor to come in and run a course tailored to your EMS. Part of the course should consist of real audits carried out by the trainees under the tutor's supervision. In this way you get your training and some auditing done for a single fee.

Before you book a course, do look at the syllabus and how long the course is. Whilst you might want to choose a more comprehensive course for your environmental manager, one day should be sufficient for a conversion course for existing quality auditors, and two days for basic environmental auditor training.

Auditor training courses

You should expect a typical internal auditor training course to include the following topics:

- An explanation of the requirements of ISO 14001.
- An overview of the most relevant legislation and aspects. (For a tailored in-house course, which of these particularly apply to you?)
- Audit scheduling.
- Planning an audit.
- Carrying out an audit.
- Writing the audit report.
- Corrective actions.
- Follow-up.

Ideally the various topics will be illustrated by case studies and practical exercises.

Standards for environmental auditing

It is worth while being aware that there is a Standard that gives guidelines for environmental auditing:

- ISO 19011: 2002 Guidelines for quality and/or environmental management systems auditing.

Any body presenting a training course will have taken these guidelines into account, but it is not really necessary for you to have copies.

Chapter 12
Assessment (Step 10)

Introduction

By now you will have carried out the following items in the project plan:

- You will have written the Register of Environmental Aspects, Register of Environmental Legislation, Operating Procedures and the Environmental Management Manual.
- The first Environmental Management Review Meeting has been held.
- The Environmental Management System (EMS) has been launched and implemented.
- Auditors have been selected, trained, and internal auditing has started.

Now is the time to choose a certification body to carry out your assessment.

Choosing an assessor

If you are already registered to ISO 9001, your first thought will probably be to go to your current assessor, who will very likely by now also be accredited to assess ISO 14001. Do not think you *must* go to the same certification body; however you will probably save money in the longer term if your quality and environmental systems are assessed by the same people. The certification bodies are trying whenever possible to dual-skill their assessors so that, when it comes to surveillance visits, one person can look at both environmental and quality systems at the same time. This will be particularly helpful if you have succeeded in integrating your systems to any extent as described in Chapters 4, 7, 8 and 14. However, because it is now straightforward to change from one certification body to another, I would recommend that you consider seeking quotes for environmental assessment and on-going surveillance of both environmental and quality systems from one or two other certification bodies as well as your existing assessor.

If you are preparing for ISO 14001 without already being registered to ISO 9001, the field is wide open.

Appendix E contains a list of certification bodies who are based in the UK and hold UKAS (United Kingdom Accreditation Service) accreditation. Do not use any assessor who is not UKAS accredited (or one of UKAS's equivalent in other countries); their certificates will not carry the UKAS logo as a seal of approval.

When making your selection, you may have a preference for a particular body because they have a particular relationship with your type of business activity. Even so, it is worthwhile getting one or more other quotes. You may be surprised at what you find. If necessary, negotiation sometimes pays off.

Quotations

Obtaining a quotation

To obtain a quotation, simply telephone your selected certification bodies and ask for an ISO 14001 Questionnaire. Fill it in, post it off and wait for the quotation. (Remember to ask the certification body to confirm that they hold UKAS accreditation for your industry sector. Otherwise they will not be able to issue the UKAS logo alongside their own.)

Comparing quotations

Quotations will state costs for application, document review, pre-visits, assessment, registration and on-going surveillance, for a three-year term. As they will all be presented in a different format, make out a table so that you can work out the total cost over three years. Look to see whether there are extras not specifically quoted. For example, some bodies include travel and accommodation within the quoted price; others will charge it as an extra and you will have to put in an allowance for this. Look at the quote for annual surveillance. Some bodies will quote an annual charge. Others will indicate the number of man-days with a day rate.

If you are concerned about cash-flow, look to see when you have to pay. Is it all up-front, do you pay as you go along, is there a payment by instalments or direct debit option?

Cost

The cost of assessment depends on the size of your organisation and to some extent on the complexity of your activities, particularly if you have any prescribed processes. The smallest organisations, up to 20–30 employees, cannot expect to pay less than about £1600. Organisations with several hundred employees could have to pay several thousands of pounds.

Document review

The document review may be undertaken on site as part of the pre-visit or at the assessor's office. He or she will be checking that your written manual and Operating Procedures appear to cover all the requirements of the Standard and that it can be understood. Any queries will be discussed with you and you can then make any necessary changes to your documents before moving on to the next stage in the assessment process.

Pre-visit

Almost certainly the quotation will include a pre-visit, sometimes called a Phase 1 assessment, when you can meet your assessor face-to-face, explain what your business does and make a tour of the site. There will be a discussion about the contents of your Registers. The visit might also include an initial audit of one or two activities. The report at the end will contain good advice, which, if acted upon, will help to make the assessment proper go more smoothly. If this option is not included, since some certification bodies choose to carry out the document review as the first day of the assessment itself, then build a pre-visit into your acceptance (and costings).

Preparing for the assessment proper

Progress

Before the assessment proper is due you should make sure that you have the following in place:

- Some evidence that you are moving towards your environmental objectives and targets. You will not be expected to have achieved them all yet, unless of course your completion date pre-dates the date of the assessment.
- A completed programme of internal audits, and also any follow-up audits where there were significant trouble spots. These are usually areas where an Operating Procedure had not been adequately implemented when it was audited the first time.
- Completion of corrective actions arising from audits and nonconformities.

The second environmental management meeting

You are advised to hold your second Environmental Management Review Meeting as soon as the results of the first round of audits are available. This time you follow the full agenda set out in model Operating Procedure 22. This is the way to bring top management's attention to any actions which need an extra push to bring them to completion before the assessor arrives.

Communication

The need for your third communication session was forecast in Chapter 5. The agenda for the session is:

- Give praise to everyone for their enthusiasm and cooperation, but only if it is justified.
- Highlight the areas that audits have shown to be troublesome.
- Describe any further work that needs to be done before the assessment.
- Stress that passing the assessment is your organisation's top priority.
- Explain what happens when the assessor arrives and comes to talk to them, and how they should respond and behave.

The script for this last point is included in the following box:

- Have you read the Environmental Policy? Can you point out where it is on display, or written down?
- Can you quickly find the copy of the Operating Procedures which apply to you? You may have your own copy, or you may share a copy with other people.
- Can you quickly find any Work Instructions which apply to the jobs you carry out?
- Have you got the right answer to the question 'What do you do when something goes wrong?'
- When the assessor comes to see you:
  - The assessor will ask straight questions. Give straight answers. They are trained not to try to catch you out.
  - If you do not understand the question, say you do not understand and ask if it can be rephrased. Assessors may use different words from the ones you are used to.
  - If you do not know the answer, say so. Do not think that because you have been asked the question you ought to know the answer; the assessor may be talking to the wrong person. If possible, direct the assessor to the right person.
  - Do not offer extra information, over and above the straight answer.
  - Show the assessor the records asked for, and no more. If possible, take papers out of a file and give them to the assessor, rather than giving the whole file.
  - Be pleasant, but do not chatter. Talking on, particularly about your problems or unnecessary details about the process or the product, will not help and may expose a weakness. This thoughtless chatter could let the organisation down.

The environmental manager's checklist

The environmental manager needs to make his or her own checks before the assessor arrives.

Carry out your own private last minute audits of:

- Document control – check that all documents are up-to-date, authorised and properly distributed.
- Training – check that everyone has had their environmental training and that the training records are complete.
- Internal audits – check that there are no overdue corrective actions.
- Management review – check that there are no overdue corrective actions.
- Calibration – check that measuring equipment used in controlling environmental performance has been listed and that calibration is up-to-date.

My experience shows that it is quite common to pick up noncompliances during the assessment in these areas quite unnecessarily, since the environment manager can, with a bit of attention, check everything is in order.

Normally you would use these last minute audits as a means of identifying and correcting minor problems and you would not write a report. However if you come across something serious which cannot be put right before the assessment, write up the audit, document the corrective action and the date when it is to be completed, which will be after the assessment. You can then demonstrate to your assessor when he or she comes across the same problem that management knows about the situation and has it under control. This should be sufficient for the assessment finding to be classified as *minor* rather than a *major* noncompliance, and so need not prejudice a favourable outcome. If the item is of truly minor importance, a fair assessor will record it as an *observation*, simply to keep it on the record so that it can be checked on the next visit.

Lastly, make sure that a signed copy of the environmental policy is on display in reception and that your receptionist knows the names of your visitors and who they are visiting.

The assessment

Looking after the assessor

Make your assessor comfortable. He or she needs somewhere quiet to work, to collect his or her thoughts, write up notes and the final report. Also provide a telephone in case there is a need for the assessor to discuss any point with head office.

Agree when there will be a lunch break and sort out the assessor's choice of menu. Assessors are accustomed to a diet of sandwiches and do not want to waste time on sit down lunches. Have plenty of coffee or tea available at other times.

The assessment timetable

Your assessor should have drafted out a timetable at the end of the pre-visit, saying when he or she plans to go on a walk-about, assess each part of the EMS, write the report and hold the opening and closing meeting.

The assessment is vital to your organisation; you want to make a good impression and make the assessor feel it is important. The managing director or other top person needs to be available and should certainly lead the organisation's team at the opening and closing meetings.

The opening meeting

The assessor will usually start by asking for a brief history of the organisation, though this may have been covered in the pre-visit. Similarly, you will be asked why you are seeking registration to ISO 14001. Even though you may be under pressure from your customers to achieve ISO 14001, this should not be the first and only reason. After all, you will have invested a lot of effort and money into seeking registration and both your organisation and the environment ought to be benefiting. Refer back to Chapter 1 for the benefit of environmental management. So go through these other aspects before bringing customers and potential customers into the debate.

Then introduce your management team, i.e. those people with whom the assessor will have most contact during the assessment.

The assessor will then recap the timetable, and the assessment will start.

The assessor's guide

Allocate a guide to each assessor. Needless to say, the guides need to know the structure of the EMS and the organisation's operations thoroughly. They have a number of responsibilities:

- To make sure the assessor does not inadvertently get into an unsafe situation. If protective clothing and equipment is needed, e.g. helmets, ear-plugs, overalls in dirty (or designated clean) areas, have a set available.

- To direct the assessor towards the right person for the subject under examination. I have known assessments get into trouble because the assessor asked a question of the wrong person who made up an answer rather than say 'Not me' and a guide who let the situation run on.

Guides must not interfere in the conversation between the assessor and the person involved. People must answer for themselves. If things go wrong for some reason, particularly if the person has made a mess of it, do not cause embarrassment by intervening then and there. Wait until you have moved away before explaining the true facts of life to the assessor.

When things go wrong

Almost inevitably the assessor will come across things which are not right. If they can be put right quickly, try to have the corrective action completed before the assessment concludes and report the fact to the assessor. It will not necessarily avoid the problem being included in the report, but the entry should be qualified to say it has been corrected.

The outcome

You have come to the closing meeting. After some words of thanks, the assessor will come to his or her findings. If your dialogue with the assessor during the assessment has been fruitful, nothing should come as a surprise. If some things were wrong, you may even have been able to put them right in the meantime.

The assessor will go through any noncompliances and observations, i.e. comments about weaknesses in or suggested improvements to the EMS. If you do not understand a noncompliance, ask for an explanation. If you accept the circumstances but are not sure that you have failed to satisfy the requirements of the Standard, ask which words in the Standard apply. Do not argue just because you feel offended because something was found to be wrong. You must retain your objectivity in what is often an emotional situation.

Noncompliances will be graded as *minor*, i.e. on the whole satisfactory but one or two items wrong, or *major*, i.e. your operation does not conform to a specific requirement of the Standard. A group of minor noncompliances on the same subject can add up to a major one.

If there is a major noncompliance you will fail and will need to discuss with the assessor how to recover the situation. This could well entail a re-visit by the assessor, at extra cost, either to repeat the assessment or just to re-examine the offending activity.

However, this should be very unlikely. You have had a pre-visit so you know your documented EMS satisfies the Standard. You will also have had other guidance from your assessor at that visit. You have audited your whole system and re-audited the trouble spots. You have communicated with your workforce throughout the project so they should be well informed.

The usual outcome is a number of *minor* noncompliances. The assessor will therefore say 'I am recommending you for registration, subject to your sending me within three weeks a corrective action plan to deal with these noncompliances'. The assessor is looking for the action plan with allocated responsibilities and completion dates; you do not have to complete the corrective actions within the three weeks.

Remember that assessors can only *recommend* registration. Their audit report is subject to review by the certification body's certification officer, whose word is final. However, assessors play it safe because they do not want you to be disappointed by someone reversing their conclusion; if they say they are recommending you, it is highly unlikely that anything will go wrong subsequently.

Surveillance visits

Your assessor will visit periodically, maybe six-monthly or at least once a year, to check that your EMS is still intact. At the first visit after the assessment, the first question will be to check that you have completed the corrective actions from the assessment. Then each part of the EMS will be re-assessed on a rolling programme spread over three years.

In environmental management systems, the assessor will on each visit pay particular attention to the environmental improvement plan. Are you setting yourself new objectives and targets each year. Are you making progress towards achieving them as planned. In other words, is the organisation steadily improving its environmental performance?

Chapter 13
EMAS

Introduction

The European Commission's Eco-Management and Audit Scheme (EMAS) came into force in 1995 as part of the European Community's policy to promote environmental sustainable development. At that time BS 7750 was operational in the UK, but there was no comparable scheme for the rest of Europe. EMAS fulfilled this function.

A number of organisations in the UK have sought assessment to EMAS, which, although initially limited to manufacturing activities and a few other sectors, is now available to any type of organisation.

The similarities

The heart of an EMS is the Registers, Procedures, Manual, auditing, corrective and preventive action, improvement and management review. These are all contained in ISO 14001, and in 1997 the European Commission accepted ISO 14001 as meeting EMAS's requirements for these parts of an EMS.

The differences

The major differences between EMAS and ISO 14001 lie in the scope of the schemes and at the start and finish of the creation of the environmental management system (EMS):

- EMAS is restricted to the European Union. ISO 14001 is international.
- Whereas the guidance notes to ISO 14001 recommend that a preliminary review should be carried out, this Initial Review is mandatory under EMAS and must be written up. The Initial Review will be verified as part of the assessment to ensure that it is comprehensive and accurate.
- When the environmental policy, objectives and targets and the management programme have been set, the organisation must produce an Environmental Statement. This must be written so that it can be understood by the public, and must include a description of the organisation's activities at the site, a quantified assessment of the significant environmental aspects, the policy and the management programme. The assessor will also check that the Environmental Statement is comprehensive and accurate. Because of the essential requirement for the Initial Review and the Environmental Statement to be independently verified, assessors who are accredited to examine applications for EMAS registration have been called 'verifiers'. Many of the certification bodies listed in Appendix E have also been accredited as EMAS verifiers.

- The Environmental Statement must be made publicly available.
- EMAS has a three-year audit cycle. ISO 14001 has annual (or more frequent) surveillance.
- EMAS places more emphasis than ISO 14001 on indirect environmental aspects, i.e. aspects that result from the organisation's interactions with third parties such as suppliers, subcontractors, customers, other stakeholders, and resulting from the use and ultimate disposal of products.

Chapter 14
Final thoughts

Integrated management systems

One of the themes running through this book is that, if you already have an ISO 9001 quality management system, many of the management functions apply to both environmental and quality systems. The coincidence of the two Standards is illustrated in Table 4.2.

The same structure has been used for more recently developed Standards for other management systems such as health and safety (OHSAS 18001). By making the structures comparable the intention is that all the different Standards should be expressed within the organisation as different facets of *one* management system.

The similarity of the structure of the three Standards is shown in Table 14.1.

If you have moved or intend to move into the paperless society, in itself an environmentally friendly decision, by creating an intranet (or internal website) for the organisation, then obviously you want a single structure. By using the hyperlink facility the user is led to the appropriate part of the system.

So, whatever the level of sophistication of your *existing* management systems, take a hard look at them before you start writing your ISO 14001 documents. See how much is common and expand that to incorporate the environmental dimension so that you only create new documents for really new topics. Keep the formats similar; it is much easier and quicker to work within an existing format rather than start afresh.

Table 14.1 Integrating management systems

ISO 14001: 1996	ISO 9001: 2000	OHSAS 18001: 1999
General requirements	General requirements	General requirements
Environmental policy	Management responsibility – commitment and policy	OH&S Policy
Planning	Planning	Planning
Implementation and operation	Management responsibility Resource management Product realisation	Implementation and operation
Checking and corrective action	Measurement analysis and improvement	Checking and corrective action
Management review	Review included in Management responsiblity	Management review

SMEs and ISO 14001

The preface to this revised edition notes that 86% of SMEs do not think that their activities harm the environment. This book is written especially for organisations such as these who want to be sure that they have taken proper account of their environmental responsibilities and who want to improve their environmental performance. Following the steps laid out in Chapter 5 should achieve this.

If you want public and certified recognition of the fact that you care for the environment, then you need to be registered to ISO 14001. Many small and medium sized organisations find this a daunting prospect. My hope is that this book with its supplements will give you encouragement and help. On the other hand, it may have had the opposite effect because of the quantity and variety of the examples given in the model Registers and model Operating Procedures. Let me try to put things into proportion.

Which environmental aspects apply to most organisations? The use of energy and water, the creation and disposal of wastes, the use of materials (including paper) and housekeeping and site appearance are almost universal. Everybody has suppliers and subcontractors. Beyond this you may have a few extra aspects. Engineering will use oils, you may create lots of traffic, your residential neighbours may be very close. For small organisations it is likely that about a dozen aspects will apply.

It is the same with legislation. Waste disposal and landfill tax, effluents, avoidance of pollution and being aware of planning restrictions can apply to everybody. Some will fall within the packaging regulations. It could be that only three or four regulations require detailed Operating Procedures in order to ensure compliance. There may be another three or four where you need to be aware that they exist but where it is unlikely that you will actually contravene them.

It is estimated that there are about 20 000 licences issued by the Environment Agency or local authorities in Britain under the Environmental Protection Act 1990. Many of these will be large organisations. Compare that figure with the fact that there are over 3.5 million SMEs in existence. It follows that only a small fraction will need detailed procedures to control prescribed processes such as are illustrated in some of the model Operating Procedures. It is much more likely that you will need to get a few basics right.

When it comes to setting improvement objectives and targets, no-one should have any difficulty in making plans to reduce energy and water usage and to improve recycling, at the very least.

Many of the organisations that are registered to ISO 9001 are small. They have successfully coped with the requirements of an international Standard. Apart from the need to carry out an initial environmental review and compile the Registers, ISO 14001 is no different.

Therefore take heart, turn back to Chapter 5, get a copy of the Standard and set to work.

Appendix A

Briefing notes for toolbox talks

As an organisation we do our best to look after and preserve the environment.

We think we can do better.

Our major impacts on the environment are . . . We need to be sure that we keep them under control and take steps to reduce their effect.

We have decided to set up an environmental management system based on the Standard ISO 14001 and to seek external registration. (This is similar to our existing ISO 9001 registration, but will require some extra Operating Procedures (and Work Instructions) to cover environmental activities.)

(Name) has been given the job of steering the exercise.

The first job will be to decide which aspects of our business impact on the environment, and to define what environmental legislation applies to us. (Name) and some others will be coming round to talk to you about the implications of your job. Please think about it in advance so that you have some ideas to discuss. You may also be asked to help write environmental Operating Procedures.

One feature of the Standard is that we are expected to improve our environmental performance. If you have any suggestions, please tell us about them.

Eventually we shall have an Environmental Management System in place. At that time I shall come and talk to you again.

Then, when the system has settled down and it has been audited, we shall invite an assessor to come and check that we are doing everything required by the Standard. (This is something you are already used to as part of our quality system.) In about . . . months' time I expect us to have our certificate on the wall.

Appendix B
Aspects checklist

You should find most of your aspects in the following list. When you have compiled your initial list of aspects, use the list to check whether there is anything you have missed.

Energy
Electricity
Gas
Fuel oil
Other fuels

Water
Water consumption: process, domestic
Effluents and composition
Drainage

Wastes
Process wastes
Maintenance wastes
Office wastes
Scientific wastes
Medical wastes
Disposal routes
Controlled and special wastes
Recycling: scrap, paper, cans, toners, etc.

Land and land contamination
Spillages
Storage
Fertilisers
Pesticides
Biodiversity
SSSIs

Emissions
Stack/vent releases: CO_2, SO_2, CO, NO_X, VOCs, other chemicals, particulates
LEVs
Radioactivity
Aerosols
Refrigerants

Transport
Mode: road, rail, etc.
Hazardous loads
Company vehicles

Neighbours
Traffic
Car parking
Noise
Odours
Site appearance
Fall-out
Community activities

Resources
Raw materials
Feedstuffs

Packaging
Packaging specifications
Quantities used
Packaging waste
Eco-labelling

Product life cycle
Resources
Manufacture
Ultimate disposal

Planning
Existing planning conditions
New developments

Suppliers
Environmental policies and practices
Subcontractors on site

Abnormal operations
Start up/shut down
Breakdown
Mistakes

Emergencies
Fire
Power failure
Spillage
Explosion
Flood
Vapour release

Appendix C
Regulations check-list

You should find that at least some of the following regulations apply to your organisations. The list is for general guidance and is not exhaustive.

Wastes

Environmental Protection Act 1990: Part II 'The Duty of Care' and the associated *Code of Practice 1996*

- Vetting of waste carriers.
- Disposal of controlled waste.
- Evidence of compliance.

The Special Waste Regulations 1996

- Disposal of special waste.
- Evidence of compliance.

Landfill Tax Regulations 1996

The Controlled Waste (Registration of Carriers and Seizure of Vehicles) Regulations 1991

- Licensing of waste carriers.

Waste Management Licensing Regulations 1994 and amendments

- On site compactors, etc. are exempt from the Regulations but have to be registered with the Environment Agency.

Landfill (England and Wales) Regulations 2002

- Landfills shall be classified: hazardous, non-hazardous, inert.
- Landfill permits specify conditions.
- Certain materials banned, including tyres, liquids, explosive, corrosive, etc.
- Closure and aftercare provisions.

Transfrontier Shipment of Waste Regulations 1994

- Need for a certificate issued by the Environment Agency to ship waste out of or into the UK, etc.

Asbestos Licensing Regulations 1983 and *Control of Asbestos at Work Regulations 2002*

- Notice must be given before carrying out any work involving the handling of asbestos.
- Asbestos wastes must be properly labelled.
- Asbestos wastes must be consigned as special waste to a designated licensed site.

Emissions

Environmental Protection Act 1990: Part 1 and the *Environmental Protection (Prescribed Processes and Substances) Regulations 1991* and subsequent amendments

- Prescribed processes.
- Evidence of compliance.

Pollution Prevention and Control Act 1999

- Redefines prescribed processes and how they are to be regulated.
- There is a timetable whereby processes already licensed under the 1990 Act are being brought into the new regime.

Notification of Cooling Towers and Evaporative Condensers Regulations 1992 and *The Prevention and Control of Legionellosis Approved Code of Practice 2000*

- Legionella.
- Control.

Clean Air Act 2000

Control of Substances Hazardous to Health Regulations 2002

- LEV maintenance.
- Helps define any hazardous substances being discharged.

Water and Effluents

Water Industry Act 1991 and the *Trade Effluents (Prescribed Processes and Substances) Regulations 1989*

- Discharges to sewer.
- The 'Red List'.
- Consent limits.
- Evidence of compliance.

Water Resources Act 1991

- Discharges to water courses.
- Consent limits.
- Evidence of compliance.

Control of Pesticides Regulations 1986

- Pesticides must be used in a way that safeguards the environment and in particular avoids pollution of water.
- Persons using pesticides commercially are required to hold a certificate of competence or be supervised by a competent person.

Nuisance

Environmental Protection Act 1990: Part III

- Statutory nuisances, e.g. noise.

Control of Pollution Act 1974 Part III Sections 60, 61 and 71

The Control of Noise (Codes of Practice for Construction and Open Sites) (England) Order 2002

Hazardous situations, processes and substances
Control of Major Hazards Regulations 1999 (COMAH) and the *Planning (Control of Major-Accident Hazards) Regulations 1999*

Replaces the *Control of Industrial Major Accident Hazards Regulations 1984 (CIMAH)*

- Hazards and risks involving the listed 'hazardous substances' must be identified.
- Emergency plans must be prepared, to the satisfaction of the Health & Safety Executive.
- There is also local authority involvement.

Planning (Hazardous Substances) Regulations 1992

- A hazardous substance consent must be obtained to permit storage of 'hazardous substances'.

Dangerous Substances (Notification and Marking of Sites) Regulations 1990

Environmental Protection (Disposal of Polychlorinated Biphenyls and other Dangerous Substances) (England and Wales) Regulations 2000 and equivalent Regulations in Scotland

- PCBs in use must be registered.
- PCBs must be removed from use and properly disposed of.

Storage
Petroleum (Consolidation) Act 1928

- No storage of more than 15 litres of flammable liquids (flash point less than 21°C) without a licence from the local authority.

The Dangerous Substances and Explosive Atmospheres Regulations 2002

- Risk assessment and appropriate risk reduction measures must be undertaken in respect of the storage and use of flammable and explosive substances, etc.

Control of Pollution (Oil Storage) (England) Regulations 2001

Transport
Carriage of Dangerous Goods (Classification, Packaging & Labelling) and Use of Transportable Pressure Receptacles Regulations 1996

Carriage of Dangerous Goods by Road Regulations 1996 and subsequent amendments

Carriage of Dangerous Goods by Road (Driver Training) Regulations 1996

Chemicals (Hazard Information & Packaging for Supply) Regulations 2002 (CHIP)

- Regularly amended, often annually.
- Gives useful hazard and risk information.

Planning
Town and Country Planning (Assessment of Environmental Effects) Regulations 1988 and subsequent amendments

Town and Country Planning (Environmental Impact Assessment (England & Wales)) Regulations 1999

Packaging

Producer Responsibility Obligations (Packaging Waste) Regulations 1997 and subsequent amendments, and the associated *Users Guide 1997* and *Ready Reckoner 1997*

- Recovery and recycling of packaging.

Packaging (Essential Requirements) Regulations 1998

- Minimum packaging consistent with product safety, etc.
- Limits on toxic metals.

Contaminated land

Environment Act 1995 Part II

- Contaminated land.

The Contaminated Land Regulations (England) 2000, also Scotland and Wales

- Definitions of types of contaminated land.
- The responsibilities, etc. for remediation.

Nature conservation

Wildlife and Countryside Act 1991 and many amendments

- Sites of special scientific interest (SSSIs).
- Protected species

Conservation (Natural Habitats &c.) Regulations 1994

- Regulation 38 ff. and Schedules list protected species.

Hedgerow Regulations 1997

- Hedgerows may not be removed without local authority approval.

Town and Country Planning (Trees) Regulations 1999

- Tree preservation orders.

Appendix D
Useful information

Standards

British Standards Institution (BSI)
389 Chiswick High Road, London W4 4AL
Tel: 020 8996 9001   Fax: 020 8996 7001
www.bsi.org.uk

International Standards Organisation (ISO)
1 Rue de Varambé, Case Postale 56, CH-1211, Geneva 20.

Environmental auditors and consultancy

Institute of Environmental Management & Assessment (IEMA)
Welton House, Limekiln Way, Lincoln LN2 4US
Tel: 01522 540069   Fax: 01522 540090
www.iema.net

(Manages the Environmental Auditors Registration Association (EARA).)

Groundwork Trade Association (National Office)
85–87 Cornwall Street, Birmingham B3 3BY
Tel: 0121 236 8565   Fax: 0121 236 7356
www.groundwork.org.uk

(Runs Groundwork Environmental Business Services, which offers environmental consultancy to large and small businesses. There are over 30 local offices throughout the UK.)

Wales Environment Centre
QED Centre, Treforest Estate, Pontypridd CF37 5YR
Tel: 01443 844001   Fax: 01443 844002
www.arenanetwork.org

(Environmental advice and consultancy in Wales.)

The Environment Council
212 High Holborn, London WC1V 7VW
Tel: 020 7836 2626   Fax: 020 7242 1180
www.the-environment-council.org.uk

(The Business and Environment Programme is an initiative of the Environment Council and assists companies to implement an EMS and corporate environment policy.)

Environmental Data Services (ENDS)
Finsbury Business Centre, 40 Bowling Green Lane, London EC1R 0NE
Tel: 020 7814 5300   Fax: 020 7415 0106
www.ends.co.uk

(Publishes the Directory of Environmental Consultants.)

Environmental advice

Environment Agency (Head Office)
Rio House, Waterside Drive, Aztec West, Almondsbury, Bristol BS12 4UD
General enquiries tel: 0845 933 3111 and 0645 333111
www.environment-agency.gov.uk/epns (for guidance information)

(Publishes Integrated Pollution Control Guidance Notes and Technical Guidance Notes for the industrial sectors which fall within the scope of integrated pollution control (IPC). Publishes Pollution Prevention Guides which apply to a number of situations. There are also videos relating to pollution prevention and waste minimisation. Advice on any situation where there is a risk of pollution.)

Scottish Environmental Protection Agency (Head Office)
Erskine Court, The Castle Business Park, Stirling FK9 4TR
Tel: 01786 457700   Fax: 01786 446885
www.sepa.org.uk

AEA Technology
www.aeat.co.uk/netcen/airqual/info/labrief.html

(Publishes the General Guidance Notes on the controls and procedures relating to environmental pollution, and the Process Guidance Notes for local authority air pollution control (LAPAC) for prescribed processes.)

Department for Environment, Food and Rural Affairs

DEFRA Helpline, Ergon House, 17 Smith Square, London SW1P 3JR
Tel: 0845 933 5577
www.defra.gov.uk

Department of Trade and Industry

DTI Enquiry Unit, 1 Victoria Street, London SW1H 0ET
www.dti.gov.uk

Best practice advice

Envirowise (formerly the Environmental Technology Best Practice Programme)
www.envirowise.gov.uk

(Publishes Good Practice Guides, Environmental Performance Guides, Case study examples and general information on a wide range of industrial sectors.)

Energy Efficiency Best Practice Programme
www.energy-efficiency.gov.uk
(Gives advice on how to reduce energy bills.)

Environment and Energy Helpline
Tel: 0800 585794
www.energy-efficiency.gov.uk

(Relates to both the above.)

BRECSU

Building Research Establishment, Bucknalls Lane, Garston, Watford WD2 7JR

Tel: 01923 664258   Fax: 01923 664787

www.bre.co.uk

(Good environmental practice in buildings.)

Construction Industry Research and Information Association (CIRIA)

6 Storey's Gate, Westminster, London SW1P 3AU

Tel: 020 7222 8891   Fax: 020 7222 1708

www.ciria.org.uk

(Good environmental practice for construction industries.)

Carbon Trust (National Office)

9th Floor, 3 Clement's Inn, London WC2A 2AZ

Tel: 020 7170 7000   Fax: 020 7170 7020

www.thecarbontrust.co.uk

(Action Energy Programme: free energy reviews, interest-free loans to invest in energy-efficient equipment. Helpline tel: 0800 585794.)

BRECSU

Building Research Establishment, Bucknalls Lane, Garston, Watford WD2 7JR

Tel: 01923 664258   Fax: 01923 664787

Appendix E

UKAS accredited environmental certification bodies

Ai Associates Limited

10 Mill Meadow Way, Etwall, Derbyshire, DE65 6NL
Tel: 01283 733 190   Fax: 01283 733 462

AJA Registrars

Court Lodge, 105 High Street, Portishead, Bristol, BS20 9PT
Tel: 01275 849 188   Fax: 01275 849 198

AMTAC Certification Services Limited

Norman Road, Broadheath, Altrincham, Cheshire, WA14 4EP
Tel: 0161 928 8924   Fax: 0161 927 7359

Amtri Veritas

Hulley Road, Macclesfield, Cheshire, SK10 2NE
Tel: 01625 425 421   Fax: 01625 434 964

Aspects Moody Certification Services Ltd

Salisbury House, Stephenson's Way, The Wyvern Business Park, Derby, DE21 6LY
Tel: 0870 752 9001   Fax: 01332 675 020

ASTA Certification Services

ASTA House, Chestnut Field, Rugby, Warwickshire, CV21 2TL
Tel: 01788 578 435   Fax: 01788 573 605

BM Trada Certification

Stocking Lane, Hughenden Valley, High Wycombe, Bucks, HP14 4NR
Tel: 01494 569 700   Fax: 01494 565 487

British Approvals Service for Electric Cables

23 Presley Way, Crownhill, Milton Keynes, MK8 0ES
Tel: 01908 267 300   Fax: 01908 267 255

BSI

Head Office, 389 Chiswick High Road, London, W4 4AL
Tel: 020 8996 9000   Fax: 020 8996 7400

BVQI

224–226 Tower Bridge Court, Tower Bridge Road, London, SE1 2TX
Tel: 020 7661 0700   Fax: 020 7661 0790

Central Certification Service Ltd

Tower Court, Irchester Road, Wollaston, Northants, NN29 7PJ
Tel: 01933 664 000   Fax: 01933 664 252

Ceramic Industry Certification Scheme Ltd

Queens Road, Penkhull, Stoke-on-Trent, ST4 7LQ
Tel: 01782 411 008   Fax: 01782 764 363

Certification International (UK) Ltd

Stratton Park House, Wanborough Road, Stratton St Margaret, Swindon, Wiltshire, SN3 4JE
Tel: 01793 829 001   Fax: 01793 829 002

Chamber Certification Assessment Services Ltd

Stowe House, Netherstowe, Lichfield, Staffordshire, WS13 6TJ
Tel: 01543 255 144   Fax: 01543 255 690

D.A.S. Certification Limited

6 Amber Court, Belper, Derbyshire, DE51 1HG
Tel: 01773 828 586   Fax: 01773 828 586

DNV Certification Limited

Palace House, 3 Cathedral Street, London, SE1 9DE
Tel: 020 7357 6080   Fax: 020 7357 6048

EAQA Limited

Office 3, Europoint Centre, 5–11 Lavington Street, London, SE1 0NZ
Tel: 020 7922 1620   Fax: 020 7922 1627

ERM Certification and Verification Services Limited

8 Cavendish Square, London, W1M 0ER
Tel: 020 7465 7369   Fax: 020 7465 7381

European Quality Assurance Ltd

Navigation House, 48 Millgate, Newark, Notts, NG24 4TY
Tel: 01636 611 226   Fax: 01636 611 704

Global Certification Ltd

1 Dovecote Close, Westminster Drive, Kettering, Northants, NN15 6GT
Tel: 01536 513 009   Fax: 01536 513 024

ISOQAR Ltd

First Floor, West Point, 501 Chester Road, Manchester, M16 9HU
Tel: 0161 877 6914   Fax: 0161 877 6915

KPMG Audit plc

Mermaid House, Puddle Dock, London, EC4V 3DS
Tel: 020 7311 1000   Fax: 020 7694 4277

Lloyd's Register Quality Assurance Ltd

The LRQA Centre, Hiramford, Middlemarch Office Village, Siskin Drive, Coventry, CV3 4FJ
Tel: 024 7688 2399   Fax: 024 7630 6055

National Quality Assurance Ltd

Head Office, Warwick House, Houghton Hall Park, Houghton Regis, Dunstable, LU5 5ZX
Tel: 01582 539 000   Fax: 01582 539 090

Rail Industry Quality Certification Limited

PO Box 464, London Road, Derby, DE24 8ZL
Tel: 01332 262 737   Fax: 01332 263 692

SGS Yarsley International Certification Services

2 Hutton Close Business Park, South Church Enterprise Park, Bishop Auckland, Co Durham,
DL14 6XG
Tel: 01388 776 677   Fax: 01388 776 691

SIRA Certification Service

South Hill, Chislehurst, Kent, BR7 5EH
Tel: 020 8467 2636   Fax: 020 8295 1990

United Registrar of Systems Ltd

United House, Station Road, Cheddar, Somerset, BS27 3AH
Tel: 01934 743 999   Fax: 01934 744 300

URS Verification Limited

Alpha Tower, 7th Floor, Suffolk Street, Queensway, Birmingham, B1 1YQ
Tel: 0121 693 3785   Fax: 0121 693 3791

Vehicle Certification Agency

1 The Eastgate Office Centre, Eastgate Road, Bristol, BS5 6XX
Tel: 01179 515 151   Fax: 01179 524 103

World Certification Services Limited

1 Bridge Road, Blundellsands, Liverpool, L23 6SB
Tel: 0151 924 7474   Fax: 0151 924 7477

Data from UKAS, as at March 2003

United Kingdom Accreditation Service (UKAS)

21–47 High Street, Feltham, Middx, TW13 4UN
Tel: 020 8917 8556   Fax: 020 8917 8499   www.ukas.com

Appendix F
Glossary

Abnormal situations	Reasonably foreseeable situations which depart from normal operating circumstances, e.g. start-up and shut-down conditions, plant failures that should be anticipated.
BS EN ISO 9001	The full reference for ISO 9001 'Quality management systems' in the UK.
BS EN ISO 14001	The full reference for ISO 14001 'Environmental management systems' in the UK.
Continual improvement	Year on year planned improvements to an organisation's environmental performance.
Controlled document	A document that must be authorised before issue, is given issue/revision status, is issued to named recipients who are automatically sent revisions and reissues and who acknowledge receipt of the document.
Corrective action	Short term action taken to overcome a nonconformity and bring the situation under control.
Emergency	A major environmental uncontrolled event often involving the emergency services.
EMS	Abbreviation for a documented 'Environmental Management System'.
Environment	Surroundings in which an organisation operates, including air, water, land, natural resources, flora, fauna, humans and their interrelation.
Environmental aspect	Element of an organisation's activities, products or services that can interact with the environment. Note: A significant environmental aspect is an environmental aspect that has or can have a significant environmental impact.

74

Environmental management manual	A description of the EMS and how it conforms to the requirements of ISO 14001.
Environmental management system (EMS)	That part of the *overall* management system that controls environmental activities including organisation, planning, responsibilities, procedures and the related documentation.
Environmental management system audit	A systematic and documented verification process of objectively obtaining and evaluating evidence to determine whether an organisation's performance conforms to the EMS.
Environmental objective	Overall environmental goal arising from the environmental policy that an organisation sets itself to achieve and which is quantified where practicable.
Environmental performance	Measurable results of environmental activity.
Environmental policy	Statement by the organisation of its intentions and principles in relation to the environment, which provides a framework for action and for the setting of its environmental objectives and targets.
Environmental target	Detailed performance requirement, quantified where practicable, which arises from the environmental objectives and which needs to be set and met in order to achieve those objectives.
Independent third party certification body	A body such as BSI, LRQA, NQA, BM TRADA, who carry out independent third party certification confirming registration to ISO 14001.
ISO 9001	The international standard 'Quality management systems' correctly known as BS EN ISO 9001 in the UK.
ISO 14001	The international standard 'Environmental management systems' correctly known as BS EN ISO 14001 in the UK.
LEV	Local exhaust ventilation equipment.
Life cycle assessment (LCA)	'Cradle to grave' impact of a product, from raw materials through processes and use to final disposal.
Management review	Periodic formal reviews by top management to ensure environmental performance is as planned and to ensure that the EMS is up-to-date and conforms to the environmental policy.
NAMAS	National Measurement Accreditation Service, part of UKAS. The body responsible for the approval of laboratories who provide calibration services.
Noncompliance	Another name for 'nonconformity'.
Nonconformity	A departure from planned activity or outcome, e.g. due to a failure to observe Operating Procedures, unforeseen circumstances, emergencies, complaints.

Operating Procedure	A statement of how an activity is managed. It states who is responsible and how the work is organised.
Organisation	A general term for any business, firm, practice, public body, etc.
Pollution	Causing environmental damage by releasing harmful substances to air, water or land.
Preventive action	Long-term actions to prevent a nonconformity re-occurring, or to prevent a potential nonconformity happening at all.
Records	The essential documents which provide evidence of actions taken, performance, etc.
Register	A statement of the environmental aspects relevant to the organisation's activities and the regulatory requirements which must be observed.
Regulatory requirements	Any legal requirement which must be observed by the organisation. In this case they relate to environmental issues and must be identified and listed.
Resources	The people, equipment and time needed to carry out a job properly.
SSSI	Site of Special Scientific Interest.
Subcontractor	Generally applied to anyone from whom the organisation purchases a service.
Supplier	Generally applied to anyone from whom the organisation purchases goods.
Tolerance	The specified range within which a parameter or value must fall.
UKAS	United Kingdom Accreditation Service. Accredits environmental certification bodies.
VOC	Volatile organic compound.
Work instruction	Detailed instructions on how to do a job. Usually displayed at the place of work.

Registers of Environmental Aspects and Environmental Legislation

A. J. Edwards

.... Ltd

Register of Environmental Aspects

Introduction

This supplement to *ISO 14001 Environmental Certification Step by Step* shows a way of presenting the Register of Environmental Aspects.

The following pages show what typical entries could look like for some of the aspects which apply to most organisations. These are followed by other entries based on real examples, which show how other types of aspects can be documented. Where numbers have been included in some of the entries to give a measure of the impact, these have been derived from real organisations. Obviously you will insert your own numbers and make your own judgements on their importance.

Take note of the comments on *severity* in Chapter 6 of the book under 'Significance of environmental aspects and legislation'. Even though you may carry out an activity every day (frequency = 3) and that activity has a high environmental impact, the scale of your operation may be so small that the severity is low when compared with that of another activity which has a lesser environmental impact but which you carry on in large quantities. The first activity, in the context of *your* organisation, may therefore rank as severity = 2, whilst the second may rank as severity = 3.

For this reason, do not assume that the significance ratings given in the following examples are absolute. You may carry out the same activity as one of those described here but in your case it may justify a different rating.

Use the 'Comment' section of each entry to record relevant findings from the initial environmental review. By doing it here you save yourself the task of writing a separate account of the initial environmental review.

If you have a number of aspects which you regard as having a beneficial impact on the environment, then the severity factors given in Fig. 6.1 and in Operating Procedure 13 can be given negative values for detrimental impacts and positive values for beneficial impacts. One educational organisation has used this to ensure recognition of the considerable effort it puts into teaching environmental subjects, recycling and creating the physical environment to promote bio-diversity. In this case the significance tables have been rewritten as follows:

Frequency of occurrence		Severity		
Description	Factor	Description	Beneficial factors	Detrimental factors
Unlikely (less than once a year)	1	Minimal environmental impact	+1	−1
Common (monthly/several times a year)	2	Low environmental impact	+2	−2
Frequent (daily/weekly)	3	Moderate environmental impact	+3	−3
		High environmental impact	+6	−6
		Severe environmental impact	+10	−10
Environmental impact = Frequency of occurrence × Severity				

Using this method would, for example, enable numerical values to be inserted in Aspect 21 Community which at present has been left blank.

To assist you in writing further entries, a blank page is included at number 23 which can be used as a template.

Each entry is cross-referenced to any related Operating Procedure and to entries in the Register of Environmental Legislation. By doing this you are making a check that you have not missed anything out of any part of the EMS.

You only need to provide the full details for aspects which are relevant to you and have a discernible impact. In your initial environmental review you may also have identified other aspects which have a negligible impact; you do not want to lose sight of these, so they are listed at the end with no supporting text. It also shows your assessor that your review was comprehensive.

The Register is available on the accompanying website. It can be downloaded and modified to suit your needs.

Contents

Register of Environmental Aspects

Issue . . . . . .   Revision . . . . . .

Dated . . . . / . . . . /200 . . . .

Page: 1 of 34

AUTHORISATION AND AMENDMENT CONTROL SHEET

Date	Issue No	Revn. No.	Page No.	Modification	Authorised by

Register of Environmental Aspects

Issue . . . . . .   Revision . . . . . .

Dated . . . ./. . . ./200 . . . .

Page: 2 of 34

1. Electricity

(Author's note: Every organisation uses electricity to a greater or lesser degree. Ways of reducing consumption usually become obvious during the environmental review.)

1. Aspect

Electricity generation consumes natural resources (oil, gas, coal) and creates atmospheric emissions CO_2, SO_2 etc. CO_2 leads to global warming. SO_2 leads to acid rain.

A kWh of electricity is equivalent to approximately 0.44 kg of CO_2.

Note the government has imposed a climate change levy of 0.43p per kWh.

2. Source of aspect

The greatest user of electricity is the factory to power plant and equipment.

Also used for lighting, office machines including computers.

3. Impact

Usage is approximately 4 000 000 kWh per annum. Corresponding CO_2 emissions are 1760 tonnes.

4. Significance

	Frequency	Severity	Impact
Normal	3	3	9
Abnormal	–	–	–
Emergency	–	–	–

5. Comment

The environmental review showed that there are opportunities to save electricity by:

- Reviewing illumination levels. Some common areas are over illuminated.
- Installing sensors in common areas so that lights only switch on when people are present and the level of natural illumination is insufficient.
- Switch-off campaign across the site but particularly in offices.
- Enabling the computer function which powers down VDUs when idle.

Register of Environmental Aspects

Issue . . . . . .   Revision . . . . . .

Dated . . . ./. . . ./200 . . . .

Page: 3 of 34

6. Operating Procedures

Operating Procedure 11   Energy control and monitoring

7. Cross-reference to Register of Legislation

13   Energy

(CO_2 emissions data from *Environmental Reporting: Guidelines for Company Reporting on Greenhouse Gas Emissions* www.detr.gov.uk/environment/envrp/gas/05.htm)

Register of Environmental Aspects
Issue . . . . . .   Revision . . . . . .
Dated . . . . /. . . . /200. . . .
Page: 4 of 34

2. Gas and gas oil

(Author's note: Most organisations use either gas or gas oil as the fuel for boilers to provide space and water heating. This example relates to an organisation which uses a gas boiler for space heating and has a process which requires a furnace fired by gas oil.)

1. Aspect

Gas and oil are natural resources and are therefore limited in the long term. Burning them generates atmospheric emissions, principally CO_2, leading to global warming.

A kWh of gas is equivalent to 0.19 kg of CO_2. A litre of gas oil is equivalent to 2.68 kg of CO_2.

Note the government has imposed a climate change levy of 0.15p per kWh for gas.

2. Source of aspect

Gas is used for the boilers to provide space heating and hot water.

Gas oil is used to fire the furnace.

3. Impact

Gas usage is approximately 210 000 kWh giving rise to 40 tonnes CO_2 per year.

Gas oil usage is approximately 60 000 litres giving rise to 160 tonnes CO_2 per year.

Spilled gas oil can contaminate land and enter the drains if not contained (see Aspect 7).

4. Significance

	Frequency	Severity	Impact
Normal	3	3	9
Abnormal	–	–	–
Emergency	1	6	6

5. Comment

Some offices and rooms are too hot. Windows are opened to compensate and then left open. Examine effectiveness of thermostat controls. Remember that a 1°C reduction in room temperature can save 8–10% of the associated heating bill.

Register of Environmental Aspects

Issue ...... Revision ......

Dated ..../..../200....

Page: 5 of 34

6. Operating Procedures

Operating Procedure 11 Energy control and monitoring

7. Cross-reference to Register of Legislation

8 Storage on site

9 Contaminated land

13 Energy

(CO_2 emissions data from *Environmental Reporting: Guidelines for Company Reporting on Greenhouse Gas Emissions* www.detr.gov.uk/environment/envrp/gas/05.htm)

Register of Environmental Aspects
Issue . . . . . .   Revision . . . . . .
Dated . . . . / . . . . /200 . . . .
Page: 6 of 34

3. Water usage

(Author's note: All organisations use water for domestic purposes. In this example, water is also used as part of the pollution control process.)

1. Aspect

Water is a natural resource. Due to ever increasing demands and periodic dry spells water shortages can occur.

2. Source of aspect

Water is used for domestic purposes.

Water to which alkali has been added is used as the entrapment curtain in the paint booths.

3. Impact

Water usage is approximately 2100 m^3 per annum.

4. Significance

	Frequency	Severity	Impact
Normal	3	1	3
Abnormal	–	–	–
Emergency	–	–	–

5. Comment

6. Operating Procedures

None

7. Cross-reference to Register of Legislation

None

Register of Environmental Aspects

Issue . . . . . .   Revision . . . . . .

Dated . . . . / . . . . /200 . . . .

Page: 7 of 34

4. Effluents

(Author's note: All organisations dispose of domestic effluent, usually to sewer. This example relates to an organisation which also uses water in one of its processes which is then discharged to sewer by permission of the local water company subject to conditions. The text also picks up the possibility of accidental spillages which can reach the site drains.)

1. Aspect

Disposal of effluents to sewer and site drains.

2. Source of aspect

- Domestic effluents to sewer.
- Contents of holding tank regularly dumped to sewer.
- Site drainage to site drains via an interceptor, and thence to river.
- Storage of solvents and oils in drums.

3. Impact

Dumping of contents of holding tank is controlled by a permission from . . . . . . Water Ltd. Dumping takes place approximately every day, up to 3000 litres (approximately 600 000 litres per annum). Any deviation from the consent conditions will constitute an offence and will upset the operations of the water company's treatment plant. This could flow through to the plant's discharge to river.

Any spillage of solvent or oils entering the site drains will ultimately pollute the nearby river.

4. Significance

Holding tank

	Frequency	Severity	Impact
Normal	2	2	4
Abnormal	–	–	–
Emergency	–	6	6

Register of Environmental Aspects
Issue . . . . . .   Revision . . . . . .
Dated . . . . /. . . . /200. . . .
Page: 8 of 34

Spillages

	Frequency	Severity	Impact
Normal	–	–	–
Abnormal	1	6	6
Emergency	1	10	10

5. Comment

The site drainage plan is kept by the Engineer.

6. Operating Procedures

Operating Procedure 6   Water treatment plant

Operating Procedure 8   Storage, housekeeping and drainage

7. Cross-reference to Register of Legislation

5   Effluents

8   Storage on site

5. Wastes

(Author's note: All organisations generate waste. In some cases it may be collected routinely by a local authority; in other cases there will be commercial arrangements with a waste carrier.)

1. Aspect

Creating waste is a waste of resources. The disposal of waste is often to landfill which is a potential land pollutant. Organic wastes in landfill generate methane which filters up into the atmosphere as a greenhouse gas.

2. Source of aspect

Wastes and rubbish generated in the office and the factory, which are not segregated for recycling.

3. Impact

...... Ltd disposes of three 8 m^3 skips of rubbish a week, 150 skips a year.

4. Significance

	Frequency	Severity	Impact
Normal	3	2	6
Abnormal	–	–	–
Emergency	–	–	–

5. Comment

The waste for disposal contains too much cardboard, which ought to be recycled. If cardboard boxes are to be thrown away, they should be flattened to reduce the volume. It should be possible to reduce to two skips per week.

6. Operating Procedures

Operating Procedure 3   Segregation of wastes

Operating Procedure 1   Disposal of controlled wastes

Operating Procedure 2   Disposal of special wastes

7. Cross-reference to Register of Legislation

1   Disposal of controlled wastes

2   Disposal of special wastes

Register of Environmental Aspects
Issue ......   Revision ......
Dated ..../..../200....
Page: 10 of 34

6. Packaging waste

(Author's note: This example relates to an organisation which receives and uses substantial quantities of packaging.)

1. Aspect

Packaging waste is a major contributor to landfill.

2. Source of aspect

Packaging discarded from imported raw materials.

Packaging used to pack finished goods for sale, which will be discarded by customers.

3. Impact

Raw materials are delivered in cardboard boxes and plastic bags with plastic sheet wrapping, amounting to approximately 145 tonnes per year.

Finished goods are packed in plastic bottles and cardboard boxes which are packed into cardboard transit packaging and palletised. Usage is approximately 500 tonnes plastic and 560 tonnes cardboard.

4. Significance

	Frequency	Severity	Impact
Normal	3	2	6
Abnormal	–	–	–
Emergency	–	–	–

5. Comment

Waste packaging was found to include new packaging declared obsolete because of a design change. The quantities in stock should be ascertained before design changes are implemented.

6. Operating Procedures

Operating Procedure 7 Packaging

7. Cross-reference to Register of Legislation

5 Packaging

Register of Environmental Aspects

Issue . . . . . .   Revision . . . . . .

Dated . . . ./ . . . ./200 . . . .

Page: 11 of 34

7. Oils

(Author's note: Many sites have diesel or heating oil storage tanks. Any organisation with a manufacturing or engineering activity will use oils.)

1. Aspect

Spilled oil can contaminate the land and enter the drains if not contained.

Waste oil is a special waste.

2. Source of aspect

Risk of leakage from storage tanks.

Engineering shop generates waste oil from bearings and engines under maintenance, waste cutting oil from machinery and oily rags, etc.

3. Impact

Heating oil storage tank holds 35 000 litres.

Approximately 800 litres of waste oil generated per annum.

4. Significance

	Frequency	Severity	Impact
Normal	2	3	6
Abnormal	–	–	–
Emergency	1	6	6

5. Comment

The oil storage tank is covered and situated in a bund whose capacity is greater than the statutory 110% of the size of the tank.

Some waste oil is being stored temporarily in various unsealed containers instead of being poured directly into the red drum. This is a safety hazard as well as a spillage risk and should cease immediately.

6. Operating Procedures

Operating Procedure 2   Disposal of special wastes

Operating Procedure 3   Waste handling and segregation

Operating Procedure 8   Storage, housekeeping and drainage

7. Cross-reference to Register of Legislation

2   Disposal of special wastes

5   Effluents

8   Storage on site

9   Contaminated land

Register of Environmental Aspects
Issue ...... Revision ......
Dated ..../..../200....
Page: 12 of 34

8. Scrap

(Author's note: Manufacturing activities usually create some metallic scrap, even if only in small quantities.)

1. Aspect

Arising and disposal of metallic scrap, e.g. steel, brass, aluminium.

2. Source of aspect

Engineering activities, e.g. machine and fabricating shops.

3. Impact

Arisings are approximately:

- 4 skips steel scrap per annum
- 1 skip aluminium scrap per annum
- 1 tonne non-ferrous scrap per annum

4. Significance

	Frequency	Severity	Impact
Normal	2	1	2
Abnormal	–	–	–
Emergency	–	–	–

5. Comment

6. Operating Procedures

Operating Procedure 3   Waste handling and segregation

7. Cross-reference to Register of Legislation

1   Disposal of controlled wastes

Register of Environmental Aspects

Issue . . . . . .   Revision . . . . . .

Dated . . . . / . . . . /200 . . . .

Page: 13 of 34

9. Housekeeping and site appearance

(Author's note: Housekeeping and the appearance of a site and its buildings applies to all organisations.)

1. Aspect

The visual aspect of the site and buildings, both externally and internally, has an impact on the environmental attitudes of all members of staff, and influences the opinions about the organisation of visitors, especially customers and regulators.

The perimeter of the site is grassed and wooded and supports wildlife.

2. Source of aspect

Actions of all staff regarding work tidiness.

Perimeter of the site is natural woodland.

Building maintenance and site improvement programme.

3. Impact

See 1 above.

4. Significance

	Frequency	Severity	Impact
Normal	3	1	3
Abnormal	–	–	–
Emergency	–	–	–

5. Comment

Noted that visual improvements to site entrance are planned in this year's budget.

6. Operating Procedures

Operating Procedure 8   Storage, housekeeping and drainage

7. Cross-reference to Register of Legislation

None

Register of Environmental Aspects
Issue ......   Revision ......
Dated ..../..../200....
Page: 14 of 34

10. Fire

(Author's note: Fire can happen to anybody even though it may not present any particular environmental risks. It should therefore be included in your Register of Aspects. This example relates to an organisation which stores flammable materials which could give rise to environmental problems if there were a fire.)

1. Aspect

Fire can release noxious smoke and particulates which will spread to the neighbourhood.

Firemen's water can become contaminated with substances released by the fire and combustion products and can enter site drains which might be overwhelmed, leading to pollution of water courses.

2. Source of aspect

Fire in any part of the site, but particularly the paint store, stocks of plastic granules, and finished goods warehouse which contains plastic mouldings.

3. Impact

Apart from the danger to life and destruction of buildings and goods, a fire could pollute the atmosphere and neighbourhood, and water could pick up pollutants and enter the site drains, overwhelming the interceptor if in sufficiently large volumes.

4. Significance

	Frequency	Severity	Impact
Normal	–	–	–
Abnormal	–	–	–
Emergency	1	10	10

5. Comment

6. Operating Procedures

(You may have an Operating Procedure to cover a fire emergency, or it may be within your health and safety system or in a separate set of emergency procedures. Cross-refer to it, wherever it is located).

7. Cross-reference to Register of Legislation

10   Major accident hazards (if your site comes under the COMAH Regulations). Otherwise refer to your health & safety system.

Register of Environmental Aspects

Issue . . . . . .   Revision . . . . . .

Dated . . . ./ . . . ./200 . . . .

Page: 15 of 34

---

11. Paper usage

(Author's note: Every organisation uses paper to a greater or lesser degree.)

1. Aspect
Paper manufacture consumes trees, water and bleaching chemicals.

2. Source of aspect
Purchases of paper for office use, computers, etc.

3. Impact
50 reams of paper equals one standard tree.

. . . . . . Ltd uses 1200 reams a year (equivalent to 24 trees).

4. Significance

	Frequency	Severity	Impact
Normal	3	2	6
Abnormal	–	–	–
Emergency	–	–	–

5. Comment
The current policy is to minimise the impact by:

- using paper derived from recyclate or managed forest, oxygen bleached.
- using the backs of non-confidential scrap paper for draft letters and reports, messages.
- printing 2-sides whenever possible.
- collecting scrap paper for recycling.

6. Operating Procedures
Operating Procedure 3 Waste handling and segregation

7. Cross-reference to Register of Legislation
1 Disposal of controlled wastes

(Paper/tree equivalence deduced from data in: Marks and Spencer plc *The Environment* 1997.)

Register of Environmental Aspects

Issue . . . . . .   Revision . . . . . .

Dated . . . . /. . . . /200. . . .

Page: 16 of 34

12. Raw materials — aluminium

(Author's note: This example relates to an organisation which uses aluminium pellets as a raw material. Raw materials in the course of their manufacture will have consumed natural resources and energy, they will have been transported possibly over long distances, the manufacturing process may have used noxious chemicals and caused or risked pollution. Some understanding of the environmental aspects of the production of your materials is desirable. This is one element of life cycle assessment. At the very least you should include in your register some comment about the environmental impact of the production of your raw materials, even if you cannot attach numbers to it.)

1. Aspect

Aluminium ore is mined, using natural resources. Mining causes damage to the local environment.

Transporting the ore from mine to smelter over long distances requires fuel. Aluminium smelting uses large amounts of electricity (approximately 13 500 kWh electricity per tonne).

2. Source of aspect

Purchase and use of aluminium pellets.

3. Impact

. . . . . . Ltd uses 200 tonnes of aluminium per annum. This will have used 2.7 million kWh electricity which will have released approximately 1200 tonnes of CO_2 to the atmosphere. Scrap aluminium is sold for re-smelting.

4. Significance

	Frequency	Severity	Impact
Normal	3	3	9
Abnormal	–	–	–
Emergency	–	–	–

5. Comment

Register of Environmental Aspects

Issue . . . . . .   Revision . . . . . .

Dated . . . . / . . . . /200 . . . .

Page: 17 of 34

99

6. Operating Procedures

(Quote here any Operating Procedures which relate to the control of aluminium usage).

7. Cross-reference to Register of Legislation

None

(Electricity required to smelt 1 tonne aluminium from www.alcan.com/Markets.nsf/Topics-E/Primary.)

Register of Environmental Aspects
Issue . . . . . .   Revision . . . . . .
Dated . . . . /. . . . /200 . . . .
Page: 18 of 34

13. Raw materials — plastic

(Author's note: This example also relates to the quantity and source of a raw material. It has been included because it notes the findings of the environmental review, as written in paragraph 5.)

1. Aspect

Plastics are derived from oil, a limited resource. The transport, refining and processing of oil carries the risk of spillage, land, sea and water pollution, and release of VOCs to the atmosphere.

2. Source of impact

Purchase and use of plastic granules.

3. Impact

. . . . . . Ltd uses 500 tonnes of virgin plastic granules per annum.

4. Significance

	Frequency	Severity	Impact
Normal	3	6	18
Abnormal	–	–	–
Emergency	–	–	–

5. Comment

Rejected plastic mouldings are granulated and mixed in controlled amounts with virgin plastic.

The reasons for the rejection of mouldings appear to be inadequately understood. A study of the causes of rejections particularly at machine set-up should produce savings.

6. Operating Procedures

(Quote here any Operating Procedures which relate to the control of plastic usage and re-use of rejected mouldings.)

7. Cross-reference to Register of Legislation

None

14. Solvent emissions

(Author's note: This example relates to an organisation which has a paint spraying process.)

1. Aspect
Emission of volatile organic compounds (VOCs) which ascend to the stratosphere and attack the ozone layer.

Any odours emanating from the site will be offensive to the neighbourhood.

2. Source of aspect
Paint is thinned with solvents. Surplus solvent evaporates in the drying oven and passes up the stacks to atmosphere.

The paint store is equipped with an extraction fan. Vapour is created during mixing operations.

3. Impact
Approximately 16 tonnes of solvent is used per annum, which is mostly released to atmosphere.

If uncontrolled quantities of solvent vapour are released and this coincides with a north wind, the nearest residents, 400 metres to the south of the site, can be expected to complain.

4. Significance

	Frequency	Severity	Impact
Normal	3	6	18
Abnormal	1	6	6
Emergency	–	–	–

5. Comment
There is an Environmental Action Plan which involves customers and the installation of new technology to change over steadily from solvent- to water-based products.

6. Operating Procedures
Operating Procedure . . .   Paint booth operations

Operating Procedure 4   Control of solvents and emissions

7. Cross-reference to Register of Legislation
3   Emissions to atmosphere

Register of Environmental Aspects

Issue . . . . . .   Revision . . . . . .

Dated . . . . / . . . . /200 . . . .

Page: 20 of 34

15. Furnace operations

(Author's note: This example relates to the use of a furnace to burn off residues as part of a drum reclamation operation.)

1. Aspect

The furnace is used to burn off residues and therefore emits principally CO_2, SO_2, particulates etc. If burning is not complete, other combustion products can be emitted, e.g. excess particulates, CO.

2. Source of aspect

Furnace stack.

3. Impact

Adds CO_2 to atmosphere (greenhouse gas), SO_2, (acid rain leading to deforestation) and particulates.

Under abnormal conditions, e.g. if the lighting up sequence is not properly carried out, smoke and odours can be emitted and cause nuisance.

4. Significance

	Frequency	Severity	Impact
Normal	3	3	9
Abnormal	2	6	12
Emergency	–	–	–

5. Comment

Under controlled conditions the furnace and stack height are designed so that combustion is complete and emissions are dispersed.

Controlled conditions means:

- Residence time minimum 2 seconds in the after burner chamber at more than 850°C.
- Adequate residual oxygen to ensure complete combustion.
- Induced turbulence to prevent cold spots.
- Gas velocity up the stacks greater than 15 m per sec.

Register of Environmental Aspects

Issue . . . . . .   Revision . . . . . .

Dated . . . . / . . . . /200 . . . .

Page: 21 of 34

6. Operating Procedures

Operating Procedure 5 Furnace operations

7. Cross-reference to Register of Legislation

4   Emissions from furnace stack to atmosphere

16. Traffic

(Author's note: All organisations generate traffic to a greater or lesser degree. The nuisance caused depends on the volume of traffic and the location of the site and its relationship to nearby residents, main roads etc.)

1.   Aspect

Traffic to and from the site can cause nuisance and pollution in the neighbourhood.

2.   Source of aspect

Employees' cars to and from work.

Lorries and vans delivering raw materials, etc.

Vans distributing finished goods.

Miscellaneous traffic.

3.   Impact

The site is on a main road 0.5 miles from the A465 trunk road. There is no housing on these roads. The nearest habitation is 400 metres beyond the site. Traffic therefore does not create a nuisance.

Number of journeys:

The site is open Monday to Friday.

Cars to site at   8.00 am   . . . per day.

                   9.00 am   . . . per day.

Cars from site at 4.00 pm   . . . per day.

                   5.00 pm   . . . per day.

Lorries and vans to and from site . per day.

average, varying between . . . . . . and . . . .

Visitors to and from site   . . . per day typical.

<table>
<tr><td>Register of Environmental Aspects</td></tr>
<tr><td>Issue . . . . . .   Revision . . . . . .</td></tr>
<tr><td>Dated . . . ./. . . ./200. . . .</td></tr>
<tr><td>Page: 23 of 34</td></tr>
</table>

4. Significance

	Frequency	Severity	Impact
Normal	3	1	3
Abnormal	–	–	–
Emergency	–	–	–

(Obviously, if the site is within a populated area, the severity and impact will be greater).

5. Comment

6. Operating Procedures
None (unless there are controls over when and how traffic moves)

7. Cross-reference to Register of Legislation
None

Register of Environmental Aspects
Issue . . . . . .   Revision . . . . . .
Dated . . . . / . . . . /200 . . . .
Page: 24 of 34

17. Legionellosis

(Author's note: Legionellosis is an environmental issue if there are 'open' cooling systems and a risk that water droplets or aerosols can be carried outside the site boundary to the neighbourhood. Remember the outbreak in Regent Street, London, which came from the BBC's cooling system on the roof of Broadcasting House. Legionella is also a health and safety issue as it can affect employees, and may be addressed procedurally in the health and safety system.)

1. Aspect
Risk of distributing airborne Legionella bacteria to the neighbourhood.

2. Source of aspect
The wet cooling tower and the main air conditioning system.

3. Impact
Can lead to death.

4. Significance

	Frequency	Severity	Impact
Normal	–	–	–
Abnormal	1	10	10
Emergency	1	10	10

5. Comment

6. Operating Procedures
(Probably in the health and safety system. May also come into 'Maintenance').

7. Cross-reference to Register of Legislation
12   Legionellosis

18. Company cars

(Author's note: This example relates to an organisation which operated a sizeable fleet of cars. Organisations which have a significant lorry fleet, either because they are a haulage company or to make deliveries, will need a comparable entry in the Register.)

1. Aspect

Cars consume petrol or diesel and generate CO_2, SO_2, NOx, particulates etc., use natural resources and cause atmospheric pollution, in particular adding to the greenhouse effect.

Tyre disposal is a major environmental disposal problem.

2. Source of aspect

. . . . . . Ltd has a fleet of 40 company cars.

3. Impact

For a typical car of 1.8 litres engine capacity, emissions would be $180\,g$ CO_2 per km. At 12 000 business miles per car per annum = 139 tonnes CO_2 emitted for the fleet.

The scale of emissions depends on how well the cars are maintained and how well they are driven.

(Note: for new cars, the cost to the organisation of vehicle excise duty is related to the vehicle's emissions index, from April 2001. The cost of the tax benefit to the user is related to the emissions index, from April 2002.)

Tyre usage depends on tyre quality and how well a car is driven.

4. Significance

	Frequency	Severity	Impact
Normal	3	3	9
Abnormal	–	–	–
Emergency	–	–	–

(Severity and impact will be related to the size of the fleet.)

Register of Environmental Aspects
Issue . . . . . .   Revision . . . . . .
Dated . . . ./. . . ./200. . . .
Page: 26 of 34

5. Comment

Driver training is included in the induction programme for new employees. Petrol consumption and tyre usage is monitored.

6. Operating Procedures

Operating Procedure 12 Company cars

7. Cross-reference to Register of Legislation

14   Company cars

(CO_2 emissions data from www.vcacarfueldata.org.uk//ved_calculator.asp)

Register of Environmental Aspects
Issue . . . . . .   Revision . . . . . .
Dated . . . . /. . . . /200 . . . .
Page: 27 of 34

109

19. Suppliers and subcontractors

1. Aspect

The suppliers and subcontractors chosen by the organisation will themselves cause environmental impacts.

2. Source of aspect

The activities of suppliers and subcontractors.

3. Impact

Some suppliers and subcontractors may have a more responsible approach to the impacts that they have on the environment, or be more environmentally aware than others.

Subcontractors working on site can be the source of environmental incidents, which will be the responsibility of the organisation.

4. Significance

Suppliers and subcontractors general

	Frequency	Severity	Impact
Normal			
Abnormal			
Emergency			

Suppliers and subcontractors on site

	Frequency	Severity	Impact
Normal			
Abnormal			
Emergency			

Register of Environmental Aspects
Issue ...... Revision ......
Dated ..../..../200....
Page: 28 of 34

5. Comment

(The significance ratings to be inserted in the above tables will derive from the information obtained about your suppliers and subcontractors in general (Procedure 10.4), and from the nature of the work being carried out by contractors working on site and the quality of their environmental management.)

6. Operating Procedures

Operating Procedure 10 Environmental aspects of suppliers and subcontractors

7. Cross-reference to Register of Legislation

None

Register of Environmental Aspects
Issue . . . . . .   Revision . . . . . .
Dated . . . ./. . . ./200 . . . .
Page: 29 of 34

20. Life cycle assessment

(Author's note: In this example an organisation shows that it recognises the theory of life cycle assessment without getting into the detail.)

1. Aspect

The impact an organisation has on the environment extends beyond those caused by its direct activities. The provision of raw materials and services will themselves generate environmental impacts. The use and ultimate disposal of the products would can also create impacts. The phrase 'cradle to grave' is often used in this context.

2. Source of aspect

Manufacture of raw materials purchased:

- The original raw materials.
- Energy used in extraction and manufacture.
- Transport at each stage of manufacture.
- Pollutants etc. released during extraction, manufacture and transport.

The organisation's activities:

- Impact of converting raw materials into finished product.

Finished products:

- Energy consumed in use.
- Ability to re-cycle when no longer usable.
- Disposal of ultimate waste.

3. Impact

Carrying out life cycle assessment (LCA) is not easy. It is difficult to define all the impacts and obtain the relevant data. It can then be difficult to decide on the relative importance of the different types of impacts to decide where the priorities lie.

4. Significance

	Frequency	Severity	Impact
Normal	–	–	–
Abnormal	–	–	–
Emergency	–	–	–

Register of Environmental Aspects

Issue . . . . . .   Revision . . . . . .

Dated . . . . / . . . . /200 . . . .

Page: 30 of 34

112

5. Comment

The organisation has decided that it does not have the expertise or available effort to carry out LCA on its existing products. However 'cradle to grave' thinking will be used when taking decisions about new products and processes.

6. Operating Procedures

Operating Procedure 14 New products and processes

7. Cross-reference to Register of Legislation

None

21. Community

(Author's note: This example relates to an organisation which involves itself in the activities of the local community.)

1. Aspect

Involvement in community activities which relate to the environment.

2. Source of aspect

Management's desire to assist the community around the site, where many employees are resident.

3. Impact

(Describe the activities.)

4. Significance

	Frequency	Severity	Impact
Normal	–	–	–
Abnormal	–	–	–
Emergency	–	–	–

5. Comment

(See the Introduction to this Register about ascribing a positive value to aspects such as this.)

6. Operating Procedures

(None)

7. Cross-reference to Register of Legislation

None

Register of Environmental Aspects
Issue . . . . . .   Revision . . . . . .
Dated . . . . / . . . . /200 . . . .
Page: 32 of 34

22. Other aspects

(Author's note: This is an example of an organisation's listing of minor aspects, which shows that the review was fully comprehensive.)

The following environmental aspects have been identified but are considered to be too minor to warrant documentation:

- Limited use of fertilisers on the grassed areas.
- Car parking space is adequate.
- Disposal of sanitary wastes.
- Arising of empty drinks cans and plastic bottles.

Register of Environmental Aspects
Issue . . . . . .   Revision . . . . . .
Dated . . . . /. . . . /200 . . . .
Page: 33 of 34

115

23. Blank

1. Aspect

2. Source of aspect

3. Impact

4. Significance

	Frequency	Severity	Impact
Normal			
Abnormal			
Emergency			

5. Comment

6. Operating Procedures

7. Cross-reference to Register of Legislation

Register of Environmental Aspects
Issue . . . . . .   Revision . . . . . .
Dated . . . . / . . . . /200 . . . .
Page: 34 of 34

.... Ltd

Register of Environmental Legislation

Introduction

This supplement to *ISO 14001 Environmental Certification Step by Step* shows a way of presenting the Register of Environmental Legislation.

The following pages show what typical entries could look like for some of the more common legislative requirements.

You will need to include in your Register all the legislation and regulations which you identified when you carried out your initial environmental review. Group them together under the activity to which they relate.

In using this supplement:

- If a page does not apply, do not mention it.
- If a page might apply at any time, include it to create and preserve awareness.
- If it does apply, then adapt the text to suit your circumstances.
- If particular legislation applies to you which is not included in the examples, e.g. countryside issues, hazardous processes, then write it up in the same format. A blank page is included at the back which can be used as a template.

Each entry is cross-referenced to any related Operating Procedures and to entries in the Register of Environmental Aspects. By doing this you are making a check that you have not missed anything out of any part of the EMS.

The Register is available on the accompanying website. It can be downloaded and modified to suit your needs.

Contents

Register of Environmental Legislation

Issue . . . . . .   Revision . . . . . .

Dated . . . ./. . . ./200 . . . .

Page: 1 of 19

AUTHORISATION AND AMENDMENT CONTROL SHEET

Date	Issue No	Revn. No.	Page No.	Modification	Authorised by

Register of Environmental Legislation

Issue ...... Revision ......

Dated ..../..../200....

Page: 2 of 19

1. Disposal of controlled wastes

1. Relevant legislation and regulations

- Environmental Protection Act 1990: Part II 'Waste on Land'
- The Environmental Protection (Duty of Care) Regulations 1991
- Waste Management: The Duty of Care: A Code of Practice (1996)
- Landfill Tax Regulations 1996
- The Landfill (England and Wales) Regulations 2002

Under the *'Duty of Care' Regulations*:

- Wastes shall be stored securely.
- Controlled wastes shall only be disposed of to a licensed waste carrier.
- All transfers of waste from the organisation to a waste carrier shall be documented on a Controlled Waste Transfer Note signed by both parties. A copy of each Transfer Note shall be kept for 2 years.
- Annual Transfer Notes can be used for regular transfers of the same waste by the same carrier.
- The Code of Practice requires checks on the validity of waste carrier licences.

Note: depending on the hazard rating of a special waste, certain proportions can contaminate controlled waste without affecting its classification as controlled waste.

The Landfill Tax Regulations:

- Disposal to landfill will be taxed at £14/t for active waste (for 2003/2004 and rising annually). General waste is active. The Government has announced an increase to £35/t in the medium to long term. Inert waste is taxed at £2/t.

Note: there is a small allowance for the contamination of inert waste by active waste without affecting its classification.

2. Relevant activities/processes
Waste arisings from the site (factory, offices, warehouse, etc).

3. Summary of requirements
Wastes are to be segregated, stored properly and disposed of correctly.

4. Procedures
Operating Procedure 1 Disposal of controlled wastes

5. Cross-reference to Register of Aspects
5 Wastes

Register of Environmental Legislation

Issue ...... Revision ......

Dated ..../..../200....

Page: 3 of 19

2. Disposal of special wastes

1. Relevant legislation and regulations

- The Special Waste Regulations 1996
- The Special Waste (Amendment) Regulations 1996
- The Special Waste (Amendment) Regulations 1997

Special wastes shall be disposed of using a five-part Consignment Note obtainable from the Environment Agency (EA) to whom a fee shall be paid.

The consignments must be pre-notified by sending one part to the office of the EA which controls the destination of the waste, to arrive at least three days before the waste is moved.

The Note shall be signed on behalf of the organisation and the waste carrier. The organisation shall keep one part (for 3 years) and hand three parts to the carrier.

2. Relevant activities/processes
Disposal of special wastes, e.g. waste oils, oily residues, solvents and sludges.

3. Summary of requirements
Special wastes shall be segregated, stored properly and disposed of correctly.

4. Procedures
Operating Procedure 2 Disposal of special wastes

5. Cross-reference to Register of Aspects
5   Wastes

<table>
<tr><td>Register of Environmental Legislation</td></tr>
<tr><td>Issue . . . . . .   Revision . . . . . .</td></tr>
<tr><td>Dated . . . . /. . . . /200 . . . .</td></tr>
<tr><td>Page: 4 of 19</td></tr>
</table>

3. Emissions of solvents to atmosphere

(Author's note: This page has been written to include text as it might apply to an organisation which falls within local authority control under the Environmental Protection Act 1990 for a Part B process. This particular example relates to paint spraying resulting in the emission of volatile organic solvents to atmosphere.)

1. Relevant legislation and regulations
- Environmental Protection Act 1990: Part 1.
- Environmental Protection (Prescribed Processes and Substances) Regulations 1991 and subsequent amendments – Schedule 1, Section 6.5 Part B(a)(ii).
- Pollution Prevention and Control Act 1999.
- Pollution Prevention and Control (England and Wales) Regulations 2000 – Section 6.4 Part B(a)(iii) supersedes the above in April 2004.
- Process guidance note PG6/23(97): Coating of metal and plastic.
- Guidance note A1: Guidelines on discharge stack heights for polluting emissions.

Organisations which operate prescribed processes require permission/licence from either the Environment Agency or the local authority depending on the nature and scale of the operation.

- Control of Substances Hazardous to Health Regulations 1999 (COSHH), Regulation 9

The COSHH Regulations require regular testing and maintenance (at least every 14 months) of any local exhaust ventilation (LEV) equipment discharging to the atmosphere.

2. Relevant activities/processes
- Spray painting: emissions of volatile organic compounds (VOCs) from the stacks on #1 and #2 paint lines.
- The paint store is fitted with an extraction system to remove solvent vapour during mixing operations.

3. Summary of requirements
Section 6.5 Part B(a)(ii) applies to paint spraying likely to release particulates and VOCs to atmosphere, with usage greater than 5 tonnes per year. . . . . . . Ltd uses approximately 16 tonnes of volatile organic solvents a year and so comes under local authority control.

...... County Council has issued an operating licence (January 1997) subject to the following conditions:

(a)   The organisation shall submit an improvement plan to change to 90% water-based paints in five years (i.e. by December 2001).

(b)   The organisation shall monitor stack emissions every three months under normal operating conditions and shall submit the results to the local authority. At no time shall the emissions of non-chlorinated VOCs and particulates respectively exceed 50 mg per m^3.

(c)   The organisation shall keep a register of quantities of solvents purchased and disposed of, and shall submit the figures to the local authority annually.

(d)   The organisation shall carry out an olfactory check daily on the eastern site boundary. If odours persist, the local authority shall be informed. A register of the daily checks shall be kept and be made available to the local authority on demand.

4.   Procedures

Operating Procedure 4 Control of solvents and emissions (for consent conditions (b)–(d))

Operating Procedure 9 Maintenance (for LEVs)

Operating Procedure 13 Environmental objectives and targets (for consent condition (a))

5.   Cross-reference to Register of Aspects

14   Solvent emissions

Register of Environmental Legislation
Issue . . . . . .   Revision . . . . . .
Dated . . . ./. . . ./200. . . .
Page: 6 of 19

4. Emissions from furnace stack to atmosphere

(Author's note: This page has been written to include text as it might apply to an organisation which falls within the control of the Environment Agency under the Environmental Protection Act 1990 for a Part A process. This particular example relates to the cleaning and recovery of drums by incineration.)

1. Relevant legislation and regulations
- Environmental Protection Act 1990: Part 1.
- Environmental Protection (Prescribed Processes and Substances) Regulations 1991 and subsequent amendments – Schedule 1, Section 5.1 Part A(d): The cleaning for re-use of metal containers . . . by burning out their residual content.
- Pollution Prevention and Control Act 1999
- Pollution Prevention and Control (England and Wales) Regulations 2000 – Section 5.1 Part A(1)(f) superseded the above in April 2003.
- Integrated pollution control guidance note S2 5.01: Waste incineration.
- Guidance note A1: Guidelines on discharge stack heights for polluting emissions.

Organisations which operate Part A processes require permission/licence from the Environment Agency.

2. Relevant activities/processes
Emissions from the furnace stack.

3. Summary of requirements
The licence from the Environment Agency:

(a) Forbids burning chlorinated residues.
(b) After burner zone to be at 850°C minimum before operations begin.
(c) Residence time of gaseous products of combustion in after burner zone minimum 2 seconds at 850°C or more for non-chlorinated residues.
(d) Induced turbulence to prevent cold spots.
(e) Adequate oxygen to ensure complete combustion (minimum 6% excess by volume).
(f) Emissions per m^3 not to exceed: particulates – 50mg; CO – 100mg; HCl – 30mg; SO_2 – 30mg; metals – 4mg.
(g) Minimum gas velocity up stack 15 metres per second.

4. Procedures
Operating Procedure 5 Furnace operations

5. Cross-reference to Register of Aspects
15   Furnace operations

Register of Environmental Legislation
Issue . . . . . .   Revision . . . . . .
Dated . . . . /. . . . /200. . . .
Page: 7 of 19

5. Effluents

1. Relevant legislation and regulations
- Water Industry Act 1991
- Trade Effluents (Prescribed Processes and Substances) Regulations 1989
- Water Resources Act 1991

2. Relevant activities/processes
- Water treatment plant treats effluents from surface treatment processes before release to sewer.
- Domestic sewage (offices, etc.) to sewer.

(Author's note: Although technically all commercial activities should have permission from the local water undertaking to discharge to sewer, licences are usually only issued where specific circumstances, e.g. the presence of listed substances, apply. It is always worthwhile including this page in your Register to show you are aware of the Acts and Regulations, but then to state in this Section 'No prohibited substances are discharged to sewer and therefore no licence is required from . . . . . . Water plc'.)

- Site drains connect to local streams and thence to the river.

3. Summary of requirements

3.1 Effluents
The following consent limits have been issued by . . . . . . Water plc:
(a) Maximum volume of effluent discharged shall not exceed 4500 m^3 per day.
(b) pH shall not be less than 5 nor greater than 9.
(c) Suspended solids concentration (dried at 105°C) shall not exceed 200 mg per litre.
(d) Chemical oxygen demand (COD) shall not exceed 6000 mg O_2 per litre.
(e) Temperature of the discharge shall not exceed 25°C.

3.2 Site drains
No oily spillages shall be allowed to enter the site drains.

4. Procedures
Operating Procedure 6 Water treatment plant
Operating Procedure 8 Storage, housekeeping and drainage

5. Cross-reference to Register of Aspects
4 Effluents

Register of Environmental Legislation
Issue . . . . . .   Revision . . . . . .
Dated . . . . / . . . . /200 . . . .
Page: 8 of 19

6. Packaging

I. Relevant legislation and regulations
- Producer Responsibility Obligations (Packaging Waste) Regulations 1997 and subsequent amendments
- Packaging (Essential Requirements) Regulations 1998

The *'Packaging Waste' Regulations 1997* apply to organisations that:

- handle more than 50 tonnes of packaging per annum, and
- have a turnover greater than £2 million.

Organisations that fall under the Regulations are required to make an annual return to the Environment Agency showing quantities of packaging in each defined category (paper, steel, plastic, etc.) at each stage in the packaging chain (raw material, convertor, packer/filler, seller), and to calculate their recovery and recycling obligations. Evidence that the obligation has been met must be provided to the Agency at the end of the year in the form of Packaging Waste Recovery Notes (PRNs).

Organisations can choose to register directly with the Environment Agency and make their own arrangements to fulfil their recovery and recycling obligations, or can join a compliance scheme which will do this for them.

The *Packaging Regulations 1997* require that:

- Product packaging shall be minimised consistent with the safe and hygienic transport and handling of the product.
- Packaging shall be designed to permit re-use or recovery.
- Printing inks shall not involve the use of heavy metal pigments.

2. Relevant activities/processes
..... Ltd falls within the scope of the *'Packaging Waste' Regulations.* The packaging involved is:

- Receipt of imported raw materials in non-returnable packaging.
- Packaging of finished goods for sale.
- Design of packaging for finished goods.

(Author's note: If your organisation is close to, but falls below, the 'Packaging Waste' threshold, you may wish to include this page in your Register, but qualify this section with the words '. . . . . . Ltd falls below the threshold and the Regulations do not therefore apply. This item is included to make staff aware of the threshold so that appropriate action is taken if the threshold is ever exceeded'.)

Register of Environmental Legislation

Issue ...... Revision ......

Dated ..../..../200....

Page: 9 of 19

129

3. Summary of requirements

...... Ltd has decided to join a compliance scheme. The scheme requires the company to:

(a) Define all relevant packaging.
(b) Keep records of quantities in each stage of the packaging chain.

4. Procedures

Operating Procedure 7 Packaging

5. Cross-reference to Register of Aspects

6 Packaging waste

7. Statutory nuisance

1. Relevant legislation and regulations

- Environmental Protection Act 1990: Part III
- Control of Pollution Act 1974: Part III Sections 60, 61, 71

Premises shall not emit any of the following, which are prejudicial to health or cause a nuisance:

- smoke
- fumes and gas
- dust, steam, smells
- accumulation or deposit
- noise.

2. Relevant activities/processes

(Author's note: Even if there have not been any complaints it is still worthwhile including this page, especially if there is a risk, particularly relating to noise or smell. One engineering company wrote the following.)

The location of the site (400 metres from the nearest habitation) means that noise nuisance is unlikely. This item has been included in the register to make staff aware of the need to control noise.

3. Summary of requirements

(If there are possible nuisances, describe them here.)

4. Procedures

(Out of the examples used in this book, Operating Procedure 4 'Control of solvents and emissions' is relevant.)

5. Cross-reference to Register of Aspects

(Similarly, Aspect 14 'Solvent emissions' is relevant.)

Register of Environmental Legislation

Issue . . . . . .   Revision . . . . . .

Dated . . . . / . . . . /200 . . . .

Page: 11 of 19

8. Storage on site

1. Relevant legislation and regulations

- Petroleum (Consolidation) Act 1928 and subsequent amendments.
- Water Resources Act 1991.
- Control of Pollution (Oil Storage) (England) Regulations 2001

Under the *Petroleum Act*, not more than 15 litres of flammable liquids (flash point less than 21°C) shall be stored without a licence from the local authority.

Under the *Water Resources Act* it is an offence to cause pollution of any water course.

Under the *Control of Pollution (Oil Storage) Regulations*, proper bunded or secure storage facilities must be provided for the storage of oil.

2. Relevant activities/processes

- Paint store.
- Storage of waste solvents and sludges awaiting removal.
- Diesel and gas oil tanks.

3. Summary of requirements

...... County Council has issued a Petroleum Licence (No P350 dated 21.01.99) which allows 600 litres of solvent to be kept in the paint store.

Waste sludges and solvents are stored in drums under cover in a concreted, bunded secure area.

The diesel and gas oil tanks are securely bunded at 110% of the capacity of the tank. The filler nozzle is within the area of the bund.

4. Procedures

Operating Procedure 4 Control of solvents and emissions

Operating Procedure 3 Waste handling and segregation

Operating Procedure 8 Storage, housekeeping and drainage

5. Cross-reference to Register of Aspects

9   Housekeeping and site appearance

Register of Environmental Legislation
Issue ...... Revision ......
Dated ..../..../200....
Page: 12 of 19

9. Contaminated land

1. Relevant legislation and regulations

- Environment Act 1995: Part III
- Contaminated Land (England) Regulations 2000 (or Scotland or Wales)

The Act places a responsibility on local authorities and on the Environment Agency to identify contaminated land and to serve remediation notices. The notices will be served on the people who created the contamination if they can be identified. Otherwise the current owner or occupier is responsible.

2. Relevant activities/processes
(Author's note: Define here if there are any concerns. These may arise from the previous history of the site or from current activities, e.g. storage and use of solvents and diesel.)

3. Summary of requirements
To prevent land contamination.

4. Procedures
Operating Procedure 4 Control of solvents and emissions

Operating Procedure 8 Housekeeping and drainage

5. Cross-reference to Register of Aspects
9   Housekeeping and site appearance

10. Major accident hazards

1. Relevant legislation and regulations

- Control of Major Hazards Regulations 1999 (COMAH)
- Planning (Control of Major Hazards) Regulations 1999

2. Relevant activities/processes
Bulk storage of propane and ammonia.

3. Summary of requirements

- Hazards and risks involving the listed 'hazardous substances' must be identified.
- A safety report must be prepared to show that all measures necessary to prevent major accidents have been taken.
- On site emergency plans must be drawn up and tested.
- Provision of information to the Health and Safety Executive (HSE) and the local authority.
- Major accidents shall be reported to HSE.
- Any proposed changes to the operations on site must be evaluated for hazards, risks and emergency plans, and submitted to HSE.

4. Procedures
Emergency plan

5. Cross-reference to Register of Aspects
10   Fire

(Author's note: If you do use and store such chemicals, you will also need an aspect relating to the possibility of leakage of vapour.)

Register of Environmental Legislation
Issue . . . . . .   Revision . . . . . .
Dated . . . . / . . . . /200 . . . .
Page: 14 of 19

11. Town and country planning

1. Relevant legislation and regulations

- Town and Country Planning (Assessment of Environmental Effects) Regulations 1988 and subsequent amendments
- Town and Country Planning (Environmental Impact Assessment (England & Wales)) Regulations 1999

2. Relevant activities/processes

- Existing planning consents
- Any future developments

3. Summary of requirements

Existing planning consents may contain environmental restrictions or requirements, e.g. landscaping, number of vehicles allowed to park on site, operating hours.

Any new planning applications likely to have significant environmental effects will require an environmental impact assessment, e.g. visual, traffic, noise, pollution.

(Author's note: Check any existing planning consents for any environmental requirements or restrictions. If there are any, then record the identity of the consent – issuing authority, date, reference number – and the nature of the requirement or restrictions.)

4. Procedures

Operating Procedure 14 New products and processes

5. Cross-reference to Register of Aspects

None

(Author's note: This is an appropriate page on which to include any nature conservation legislation, if it applies.)

Register of Environmental Legislation

Issue ...... Revision ......

Dated ..../..../200....

Page: 15 of 19

12. Legionellosis

1. Relevant legislation and regulations

- Control of Substances Hazardous to Health Regulations 1999 (COSHH)
- Notification of Cooling Towers and Evaporative Condensers Regulations 1992
- The control of legionella bacteria in water systems. Approved Code of Practice and guidance. HSE (L8) 2000.
- Legionnaire's disease. A guide for employers. HSE (L27) 2000.

If a site has a wet cooling tower or an evaporative condenser open to the atmosphere, the local authority must be informed and steps taken to prevent or control the growth of the Legionella bacterium.

(Author's note: See the introduction to Aspect 17.)

2. Relevant activities/processes
The cooling tower and the main air conditioning system.

3. Summary of requirements

- System cleaned and disinfected in spring and autumn, and before recommissioning if it has been taken out of use.
- Make-up water to be dosed with scale and corrosion inhibitors, dispersants and biocides.
- Monthly test of water quality.

4. Procedures
(Probably in the health and safety system. Make sure the procedure includes dealings with the local authority. May also come into 'Maintenance'.)

5. Cross-reference to Register of Aspects
17   Legionellosis

Register of Environmental Legislation

Issue ...... Revision ......

Dated ..../..../200....

Page: 16 of 19

13. Energy

1. Relevant legislation and regulations

- Finance Bills 1999 and 2000

As one action to meet the Kyoto commitment to reduce emissions of greenhouse gases, HM Government announced a climate change levy or carbon energy tax on the industrial and commercial use of energy to apply from April 2001, exempting energy from new forms of renewable energy, e.g. solar, wind power.

2. Relevant activities/processes

Applies to all energy used by . . . . . . Ltd.

3. Summary of requirements

Current levy is 0.15p per kWh for coal and gas, 0.07p per kWh for LPG, and 0.43p per kWh for electricity (at March 2003).

4. Procedures

Operating Procedure 11 Energy control and monitoring

5. Cross-reference to Register of Aspects

1 Electricity
2 Gas and gas oil

Register of Environmental Legislation

Issue . . . . . .   Revision . . . . . .

Dated . . . . / . . . . /200 . . . .

Page: 17 of 19

14. Company cars

1. Relevant legislation and regulations

- Finance Bill 2000

2. Relevant activities/processes

Administration of the fleet of company cars.

3. Summary of requirements

From April 2001 the basis for charging Vehicle Excise Duty on new passenger vehicles is related to the vehicle's CO_2 emissions.

4. Procedures

Operating Procedure 12 Company cars

5. Cross-reference to Register of Aspects

18   Company cars

Register of Environmental Legislation
Issue . . . . . .   Revision . . . . . .
Dated . . . . / . . . . /200 . . . .
Page: 18 of 19

15. Blank

1. **Relevant legislation and regulations**

2. **Relevant activities/processes**

3. **Summary of requirements**

4. **Procedures**

5. **Cross-reference to Register of Aspects**

Operating Procedures

A.J. Edwards

Introduction

These model Operating Procedures have been written to give guidance on ways in which different aspects of an environmental management system (EMS) can be managed. If you already have your own way of controlling some of them, stay with what you have got, but do check that you have addressed *all* the relevant requirements of ISO 14001.

There are so many possible environmental aspects that it would have been difficult to have provided a model procedure for every one. I hope that some of the examples may be directly relevant to your organisation. If not, I hope that they give you enough guidance so that you can write your own procedures to control other aspects that you have identified as part of your own environmental management programme. The texts included here also address the legislation that is commonly found to apply to most organisations and to give examples of procedures that address some of the other legal requirements that may apply to you. Lastly there are the procedures dealing with the specific administrative requirements of ISO 14001. The link between these procedures and the clauses of the Standard is recorded in the model Environmental Management Manual.

The model Operating Procedures fall into the above categories, as follows:

- Observing the law: 1, 2, 4–9.
- Managing environmental aspects: 3–6, 8, 10–12, 14.
- Managing the EMS: 9, 10, 13–22.

So, select which models you need from the first two groups and write your own procedures for any other legal requirements or environmental aspects that apply to you. Then make sure that you have procedures to deal with all the topics in the third group. If you are registered to ISO 9001 you will find you have existing procedures that deal with some of the requirements which can be expanded to bring in the environmental dimension; the model Operating Procedures are annotated to show where this should be possible.

You will notice that the model procedures do not have title pages or amendment control sheets. Title pages are unnecessary. Putting an amendment control sheet on each copy of the procedures is also unnecessary; the environmental manager can put a control sheet on the master copy so that the history of each Operating Procedure can be traced. By making these changes from what is a common practice you will save two sheets of paper for every procedure distributed; you can work out the environmental gain.

When using the models, you will obviously incorporate your own job titles and allocated responsibilities. Suggestions are made, and possible alternatives are shown (OR . . . . . .). The same technique is used where alternative texts have been included.

The word 'organisation' has been used throughout to describe your business, firm or company. I suggest you change this to 'company', 'firm', 'practice', etc. as this will give a greater sense of identity to the users of the procedures. Where '. . . . . . Ltd' is written, I suggest you insert the actual name of your organisation.

All the model procedures are based on real life examples and can be freely adapted to suit your circumstances. They are available on the accompanying website. They can be downloaded and modified as required.

Index of Operating Procedures

Operating Procedure No. 1

Disposal of controlled wastes

1. Purpose and scope

This procedure ensures that only licensed waste carriers are used to remove wastes, and that disposals of controlled waste are correctly documented as required by the *Environmental Protection Act 1990: Part II 'The Duty of Care'*, and *Waste Management: The Duty of Care: A Code of Practice (1996)*.

2. Responsibility

The Environmental Manager (OR Purchasing Manager OR ......) is responsible for selecting waste carriers and checking that they have a valid carrier's licence.

The Environmental Manager (OR Security staff OR ......) is responsible for signing and receiving Controlled Waste Transfer Notes when waste is removed.

The Environmental Manager (OR ......) is responsible for filing Transfer Notes.

3. Checking waste carrier licences

3.1 Checking

Before placing an order or a contract with a waste carrier, the carrier shall be asked to provide a copy of his Waste Carrier Licence.

Check with the issuing office of the Environment Agency that the licence is still valid. This can be done by telephone.

The local office of the Environment Agency is at: (insert address)

Telephone: (insert telephone number)

For other areas, use the Agency's general enquiry line 0845 933 3111 (local call rate) to ask for the relevant telephone number.

Record the fact of the check on the copy licence.

3.2 Exceptions

Note that the local Council is not required to hold a waste carrier's licence for its own waste carrying activities.

Note that charities can be exempted from the requirement to hold a licence. Check that they have officially obtained an exemption.

Operating Procedure 1:   Issue ......

Dated ..../..../200....

Page: 1 of 3

3.3 Filing
Licences shall be filed by the Environmental Manager (OR . . . . . .).

3.4 Annual check
There shall be an annual check with the Environment Agency that licences are still valid. The outcome of the check shall be recorded on the copy licence.

3.5 Expiry of licences
New copy licences shall be obtained when a licence expires.

4. Disposal of controlled waste

4.1 Definition
Controlled waste includes all wastes produced by . . . . . . Ltd except 'special waste' as defined in Operating Procedure 2 (mainly oils, solvents, sludges, ...).

4.2 Controlled Waste Transfer Notes
All transfers of waste shall be documented on a Controlled Waste Transfer Note. Any member of staff responsible for handing over waste to a Waste Carrier must sign a Transfer Note, unless an annual Transfer Note (see paragraph 4.3) is in effect.

The Note is normally provided by the Waste Carrier. If no Transfer Note is available, the form in Annex A can be photocopied.

(Author's note: It is the organisation's responsibility to provide the Transfer Note, but usually the waste carrier provides his own documentation. It is advisable to have spare Notes available in case the driver is empty handed. There is a recommended form in the Code of Practice book which you can append as your Annex A.)

4.3 Annual (or period) Transfer Notes
The Environmental Manager (OR . . . . . .) shall decide whether to document all regular transfers for up to a 12-month period on an annual Transfer Note.

All transfers using an annual Transfer Note must be:

- the same category of waste
- to the same Waste Carrier
- transferred at the same location.

4.4 Transfer Note information
Transfer Notes shall contain the following information:

- Description of the waste
- How it is contained
- Quantity – which can be in units such as skips, sacks, drums
- Name and address of . . . . . . Ltd
- Name and address of the waste carrier

> Operating Procedure 1:   Issue . . . . . .
>
> Dated . . . ./. . . ./200. . . .
>
> Page: 2 of 3

- The waste carrier's registration number
- The address where the transfer took place
- Date of the transfer (or start and finish date for multiple transfers)
- Signed by the organisation's representative
- Signed by the representative of the waste carrier, e.g. the driver.

4.5 Records

Completed Transfer Notes shall be filed and retained for two years from the date of expiry.

Operating Procedure 1:   Issue . . . . . .

Dated . . . . / . . . . /200 . . . .

Page: 3 of 3

Operating Procedure No. 2

Disposal of special wastes

1. Purpose and scope
This procedure ensures that disposals of special wastes are managed in conformity with the requirements of *The Special Waste Regulations 1996*.

2. Responsibility
The Environmental Manager (OR . . . . . .) is responsible for identifying special wastes arising on site.

If any member of staff is concerned that a waste might be special waste, he or she shall refer to the Environmental Manager (OR . . . . . .).

The Environmental Manager (OR . . . . . .) is responsible for arranging removals of special waste, and preparing and signing, and filing Special Waste Consignment Notes.

3. Definitions
The definition of special waste is given in the Regulations. In general terms, it includes wastes which are highly flammable, harmful, toxic, irritant, corrosive.

The following wastes produced by . . . . . . Ltd have been classified as special waste:

- Waste oil
- Waste solvents and paint residues
- Chemicals.

Guidance is given in *Special wastes: a technical guidance note on their definition and classification (HMSO 1999)*. Hazardous properties for chemical products can be obtained from the *Chemicals (Hazard Information and Packaging for Supply) Regulations 2002 (CHIP)* as amended.

4. Disposal of special waste

4.1 Waste carriers
Waste carriers shall be selected as described in Operating Procedure 1 'Disposal of controlled wastes'.

4.2 Obtaining a Consignment Note
Disposals of special waste are controlled using a Special Waste Consignment Note.

Standard Consignment Notes can be obtained from the Environment Agency, or may be supplied on your behalf by the waste carrier.

Operating Procedure 2:   Issue . . . . . .
Dated . . . . /. . . . /200. . . .
Page: 1 of 3

If you need to obtain a Consignment Note:

- For 20 notes or less, contact or visit the local area office of the Environment Agency: (insert address and telephone number). If Notes are collected in person, the £15 fee is payable directly.
- For more than 20 notes, contact the Peterborough office: Environment Agency, PO Box 398, PETERBOROUGH PE2 5DW, Tel: 0354 001166 (local call rate), Fax: 01 733 358172

If notes are sent by post, they will be invoiced. These Consignment Notes are pre-coded.

The Waste Carrier's design of Consignment Note can be used, provided it contains all the relevant information. Before using a note, obtain a code number from the Peterborough office. This can be done by telephone. This will trigger the invoicing procedure.

4.3 Completing a Consignment Note

When making a disposal, using the five part set:

- Before moving the consignment, prepare Parts A and B of the note and enter the code number. Send the first sheet (white) to the agency office covering the area in which the recipient of the waste is located. If in doubt which office to use, ring the Environment Agency's enquiry number 0645 333111 (local call rate).
- When making the despatch, complete Part C of the note with the carrier's details. Both the Environmental Manager (OR ......) and the carrier's representative (e.g. the driver) shall sign the note.

Keep the green copy, and hand the other three copies to the carrier.

(In due course, one of these copies will be returned to the Environment Agency, who will match it to the pre-notification copy.)

4.4 Multiple consignments

If the same type of special waste is to be disposed of by the same carrier in a period of time, up to one year, the multiple consignment procedure can be used.

If there are going to be multiple consignments of the same type of special waste, only the **first** consignment need be pre-notified. The Consignment Note should be endorsed in Part A to indicate that there will be further consignments. Part B should give an indication of the total amount of waste to be moved (e.g. disposing of 100 tonnes of material in 20 tonne loads).

For each **successive** consignment, discard the pre-notification (white) copy of the Consignment Note set and complete the rest of the documentation as above, making a note on the Consignment Note that it is part of a series of consignments.

Operating Procedure 2: Issue ......

Dated ..../..../200....

Page: 2 of 3

Note: The Consignment Note will carry its own code number. You must also write on the code number of the first consignment.

Fees are payable per Consignment Note, i.e. payment per load.

4.5 Exceptions
There are some exceptions to the above procedures:

Lead batteries:	For disposals of lead batteries, pre-notification is not required. Discard the pre-notification copy of the Consignment Note set. The fee is £10.
Carrier's round:	There are special provisions where a carrier collects the same type of waste from specified consignees and delivers it to a single destination.
Other:	There are other variations, such as where off-specification products are being returned to their manufacturer, transfers are between locations in the same group for storage purposes.

4.6 Filing
Completed Consignment Notes shall be filed in the Waste Transfer Note file which acts as the register.

Consignment Notes shall be retained for three years from the date of expiry.

Operating procedure No. 3

Waste handling and segregation

1. Purpose and scope

This procedure sets out how wastes that arise across the site shall be segregated and stored so that recovery and recycling can be maximised and the correct disposals made.

2. Responsibility

All staff are responsible for the correct handling, segregation and storage of waste materials.

Operators in goods inwards are responsible for processing waste plastic sheet.

Operators in the reprocessing area are responsible for emptying rejected bottles of product.

The fork truck driver and labourers are responsible for moving waste containers to the yard, ready for collection.

Office staff are responsible for the segregation of office wastes.

Cleaners are responsible for removing office wastes.

The Purchasing Department, Yard Foreman and Storeman are responsible for the disposal of wastes.

Operating Procedure 3:   Issue . . . . . .

Dated . . . . / . . . . /200 . . . .

Page: 1 of 5

3. Factory

3.1 Waste segregation

Waste arisings shall be segregated at the point of arising and stored as follows:

Ferrous scrap	Yellow skips
Ferrous swarf	Blue bins
Non-ferrous metals	White bins
Cardboard boxes	To be flattened and stacked on pallets
Waste oils	Red drums
Oily rags	Red bins
Plastic sheet packaging	To be de-labelled and baled (see 3.2 below)
Pallets	Stacked
Reject bottles, including bottles filled with product	Cages (see 3.4 below)
General rubbish	Black bins

3.2 Waste plastic sheet packaging

There are scissors at the baling station. All labels shall be removed from the plastic sheet and disposed of as rubbish.

The plastic sheet shall be placed in the wall-mounted baler. When the baler is full, the piston shall be pulled down to create bales.

Operating Procedure 3:   Issue . . . . . .

Dated . . . . / . . . . /200 . . . .

Page: 2 of 5

3.3 Waste handling in the factory

Waste containers when full shall be moved to:

Yellow skips (ferrous scrap)	Empty into large yellow skip (yard)
Blue bins (ferrous swarf)	Empty into large swarf skip (yard)
White bins (non-ferrous materials)	Skip in stores
Pallets of cardboard	Strap. Move to despatch area in stores.
Red drums (waste oils). Red bins (oily rags)	To be sealed. Store in the covered bunded area.
Bales of plastic film	Stack on pallets. Strap. Move to despatch area in stores.
Stacked pallets	To designated area (yard)
Cages of reject bottles from factory	To reprocessing area
Cages of reject bottles from reprocessing area (see 3.4 below)	Move to despatch area in stores.
Drums of reject product	To be sealed. Store in the covered bunded area.
General rubbish	Covered skip

3.4 Reject bottles of product – reprocessing area

The contents of bottles shall be poured into drums. The drums shall be sealed and labelled.

The empty bottles shall be caged, ready for disposal.

4. Offices

4.1 Waste segregation

Clean waste paper	Octabins
Toner cartridges	Box by photocopier
General rubbish	Waste bins

4.2 Waste handling

Waste paper	To designated covered skip (yard)
Toner cartridges	Collected by service engineer
General rubbish	Covered skip

5. Disposal

The Yard Foreman and Storeman shall advise the Purchasing Department when bins, skips, etc. are ready for disposal.

The Purchasing Department shall make arrangements with contractors for the removal of wastes (see Operating Procedure 1 'Disposal of controlled wastes' and Operating Procedure 2 'Disposal of special wastes').

6. Work Instructions

(Author's note: This is an ideal application for the use of Work Instructions. For example, the table in paragraph 3.1 can be enlarged and displayed at key points in the factory. Paragraph 3.2 can be displayed at the baler. Paragraph 3.3 can be in the fork truck driver's cabin, etc.)

Operating Procedure 3:   Issue . . . . . .
Dated . . . . / . . . . /200 . . . .
Page: 4 of 5

Operating Procedure No. 4

Control of solvents and emissions

(Author's note: This procedure is based on an example of a paint spraying process which comes under local authority control.)

1. Purpose and scope

This procedure describes the actions which shall be taken to ensure that solvents and solvent emissions are controlled and satisfy the consent conditions laid down by ...... County Council under the *Environmental Protection Act 1990: Part 1.*

2. Responsibility

The Environmental Manager has overall responsibility for records relating to solvent use and emissions and for communications with the local authority.

The Environmental Manager shall arrange for the sampling of stack emissions, sending solvent sludges for recovery and disposal, and for calculations of weight of solvent released to atmosphere.

The Paint Technician is responsible for paint store operations and for keeping a register of solvent purchased, used, despatches of waste solvent and stocks.

The Plant Manager is responsible for investigating and taking corrective action if emissions are found to breach the consent limits.

Security staff are responsible for the daily olfactory check, keeping the Solvent Odour Book and alerting the Environmental Manager if significant odours have been released.

3. Consent conditions

The following conditions have been laid down by the local authority:

(a) Monitor emissions from stacks on #1 and #2 paint lines every three months under normal operating conditions and submit results to local authority. Emissions of non-chlorinated VOCs and particulates shall not exceed $50\,mg$ per m^3 respectively.
(b) Keep a register of solvent purchased and disposed of. Submit figures to local authority annually.
(c) Daily olfactory checks on eastern site boundary. If odour persists inform local authority. Keep a register of checks, to be available on demand.

Operating Procedure 4:   Issue ......

Dated ..../..../200....

Page: 1 of 3

---

4. Stack emissions

Every three months, an approved sub-contract laboratory shall sample the emissions on stacks #1 and #2 when the paint lines are working normally.

Copies of the results shall be submitted to the local authority.

If the emissions of VOCs or particulates exceed 50 mg per m^3, re-sampling shall take place. If the problem persists an Environmental Nonconformance/Incident Report shall be written and sent to the Environmental Manager. The Plant Manager shall investigate the operating conditions and take corrective action to bring the emissions back under control.

5. Solvent Register

The Plant Technician shall keep a Register of solvents purchased, solvents used, and waste solvents sent for recovery.

Sludge residues shall be sent for recovery. The contractor shall be required to advise . . . . . . Ltd of the quantity of solvent recovered. This shall be entered into the Register.

There shall be a stock take and balancing of the Register every three months to calculate the approximate weight of solvent released to atmosphere.

6. Paint store operations

All mixing operations shall take place within the paint store and within the area of the floor bund. Diluted paint for use shall be transferred to the paint lines in the sealed containers ready to be attached to the paint inlet pipe.

Any paint or spillage shall be sucked up and placed in empty drums. Any absorbent medium used shall be placed in drums. The drums shall be sealed.

Empty drums shall be sealed.

Empty drums and drums holding waste solvent or sludges shall be kept under cover in the covered, locked and bunded compound.

Paint or solvent must not be allowed to spill onto the concrete yard surface or the surrounding gravel areas.

7. Odour releases

The morning duty Security Officer shall daily on his first round when the plant is operating visit the eastern boundary and check for solvent odour in the air.

The fact of the check and the findings (no smell, faint, noticeable or strong smell) shall be recorded in the Solvent Odour Book kept in the Security office.

If any smell is detected the Plant Manager shall be informed, who shall investigate the cause and take corrective action.

Operating Procedure 4:   Issue . . . . . .

Dated . . . . / . . . . /200 . . . .

Page: 2 of 3

If the smell is noticeable or strong, the Environmental Manager shall also be informed. The incident shall be recorded on an Environmental Nonconformance/Incident Report. The Environmental Manager shall decide whether to inform the local authority.

(Author's note: This company would also have an operating procedure for the paint lines. As an example of how to make people aware of the environmental implications of their jobs, the following words would be included in the procedure 'Paint spraying shall not start until the water curtain has been dosed and is circulating properly. Otherwise, paint and solvent vapour will escape up the stacks to atmosphere, contravening the local authority's licence conditions and causing a smell nuisance which will result in complaints from the community. Paint spraying shall stop immediately if water circulation is interrupted'.)

Operating Procedure No. 5

Furnace operations

(Author's note: this procedure is included to show that starting up (or shutting down) a process is a time when there is a greater risk of an environmental incident than when the process is operating normally.)

1. Purpose and scope

This procedure ensures that furnace operations at start up, normal operations and shut down are controlled and satisfy the consent conditions laid down by the Environment Agency under the Pollution Prevention and Control Act 1999.

2. Responsibility

Furnace operators are responsible for operating the furnace correctly in accordance with this procedure.

3. Consent conditions

(a) Only non-chlorinated residues shall be processed.
(b) Residence of gaseous products of combustion in after burner zone 2 seconds minimum at 850°C minimum.
(c) Adequate oxygen for complete combustion.
(d) Induced turbulence to prevent cold spots.
(e) Emissions per m^3 not to exceed: particulates – 50 mg; CO – 100 mg; HCl – 30 mg; SO_2 – 30 mg; metals – 4 mg.
(f) Gas velocity up stack 15 metres per second minimum.

This procedure applies to (b)–(d).

4. Operations

4.1 Start-up

The conveyor shall be empty before the furnace is lit.

The normal burners shall be lit in the pre-heat and combustion zones.

When the furnace temperature in the combustion zone reaches 750°C, the after burners shall be lit and the fan switched on.

When the temperature in the after burner zone reaches 860°C and has held for five minutes, drums shall be fed onto the conveyor. Feed rate not to exceed 120 drums per hour.

The temperature and fan alarms shall be switched on.

Operating Procedure 5:   Issue ......
Dated .... / .... /200 ....
Page: 1 of 2

4.2 Normal operations

The alarm will trigger if the temperature drops below 855°C. The fan alarm will trigger if the fan stops. If this happens, the conveyor shall be stopped until the operating temperature of 860°C has been restored.

4.3 Shut down

The conveyor shall be cleared of all drums before the furnace is switched off.

4.4 Environmental impact

IF DRUMS ARE PROCESSED WHEN THE FURNACE IS NOT UP TO TEMPERATURE, BLACK SMOKE AND UNBURNT RESIDUES (SMELLS) WILL BE EMITTED. THIS WILL CONTRAVENE OUR OPERATING LICENCE, WILL LEAD TO COMPLAINTS AND COULD LEAD TO US BEING PROSECUTED OR SHUT DOWN.

Operating Procedure 5:   Issue . . . . . .

Dated . . . ./. . . ./200 . . . .

Page: 2 of 2

Operating Procedure No. 6

Water treatment plant

(Author's note: This procedure is based on an example where a consent to discharge effluents is required. The licence would be issued by the water company unless the site falls within the scope of the Pollution Prevention and Control Act 1999 (PPC)) when it would be issued by the Environment Agency.)

1. Purpose and scope

This procedure describes the operations of the water treatment plant, to ensure that effluent discharged from the site is within the consent conditions laid down by . . . . . . Water plc.

2. Responsibility

The Technical Manager has overall responsibility of water treatment, and also monitors the operation and investigates if it appears the analysis of untreated effluent is going out of control.

The Water Treatment Supervisor has day-to-day control of water treatment.

The Operator carries out sampling, analytical and dosing activities, and keeps records.

The Technical Manager or Water Treatment Supervisor is responsible for alerting . . . . . . Water plc if there is any release that breaches the consent conditions.

3. Consent conditions

The consent conditions are:

(a) Maximum volume of effluent discharged shall not exceed $4500\,m^3$ per day.
(b) pH shall not be less than 5 nor greater than 9.
(c) Suspended solids concentration (dried at 105°C) shall not exceed $200\,mg$ per litre.
(d) Chemical oxygen demand (COD) shall not exceed $6000\,mg\,O_2$ per litre.

Temperature of the discharge shall not exceed 25°C.

4. Operations

4.1 Collection of effluent

Process effluents tend to be acidic.

Process effluents are collected via a collection chamber into the holding tank. When the holding tank is three quarters full the input valve shall be closed and the liquid shall be sampled and analysed for pH, suspended solids and COD.

4.2 pH control

If pH is less than 5, use the Dosing Table to determine the quantity of 25% sodium hydroxide solution to add. Resample. Aim for pH 6 but in the range 5–9.

Operating Procedure 6:   Issue . . . . . .

Dated . . . . /. . . . /200. . . .

Page: 1 of 2

162

4.3 Suspended solids and COD control

If suspended solids exceed 200 mg per litre and/or COD exceeds 6000 mg O_2 per litre, use the Dilution Tables to determine how much water to add. Resample.

4.4 Release

Check temperature. If in excess of 25°C, hold until temperature drops. Then release to sewer.

5. Records

All sampling results and corrective actions taken shall be recorded in the Log Sheet.

6. Breach of consent limit and emergencies

If effluent is released which breaches the consent limit, the Supervisor or Manager shall be informed immediately. The Supervisor or Manager shall report the incident to . . . . . . Water plc without delay.

An Environmental Nonconformity/Incident Report shall be written and sent to the Environmental Manager.

7. Precautions

During collection of effluent into the holding tank, the outlet valve must be shut.

During sampling and adjustment of the contents of the tank all valves must be shut.

During discharge, the inlet valve must be shut.

During maintenance all valves must be shut, and returned to normal when the plant is handed back to operatives.

The inlet and outlet valves must never both be open at the same time – this would allow un-sampled untreated effluent to flow into the sewer, which could breach the consent limits and lead to the organisation being prosecuted.

8. Monitoring Operations

Log Sheet records shall be analysed to look for trends in the analysis of untreated process effluents. If the effluents are tending to be too acidic and the analysis has to be corrected frequently, there shall be an investigation into the processes and their operating parameters.

9. Work Instructions

Sampling and analysis method for pH

Sampling and analysis method for suspended solids

Sampling and analysis method for COD

Dosing Table – pH

Dilution Table – suspended solids

Dilution Table – COD

Operating Procedure No. 7

Packaging

(Author's note: This model Operating Procedure has been written for an organisation that carries out the following activities. The tables will have to be adapted to suit your activities.

- *Raw materials, some imported, are converted into a product which is packed into plastic bags. The bags are boxed and palletised.*
- *Some product goes directly to UK end-users; some goes to UK distributors for onward sale; some is exported.*
- *Sales of manufactured product are boosted by purchasing some finished product ready packed from both UK sources and imports for onward sale.)*

1. Purpose and scope

. . . . . . Ltd falls within the scope of the '*Producer Responsibility Obligations (Packaging Waste) Regulations 1997*'.

This procedure ensures that the data required by the (name) compliance scheme (OR the Environment Agency) is defined and provided at the correct time.

2. Responsibility

The Environmental Manager (OR . . . . . .) has overall responsibility for ensuring that packaging data is collected and processed and that returns are made to the (name) compliance scheme (OR the Environment Agency) by the due date.

The Purchasing Manager (OR . . . . . .) shall obtain data on the weights of packaging from suppliers.

The Accountant (OR IT Manager OR . . . . . .) shall set up the invoicing system so that it can collect data on packaging weights despatched.

3. Types of packaging

The following packaging has been identified:

	Paper (inc cardboard)	Plastic	Glass	Steel	Aluminium	Wood
Imported raw materials	✓	✓	–	–	–	✓
Strapping on imported goods	–	–	–	✓	–	–
Finished goods primary packaging	✓	✓	–	–	–	–
Finished goods transit packaging	✓	–	–	–	–	–
Pallets for finished goods	–	–	–	–	–	✓
Strapping on finished goods	–	✓	–	–	–	–

Operating Procedure 7:   Issue ......

Dated ..../..../200....

Page: 2 of 5

4. Summary of packaging obligations

The following categories of packaging incur an obligation as shown:

	Raw materials	Convertor	Packer/ filler	Seller
Imported raw materials	✓	✓	✓	✓
Imported purchased products for direct sale to UK end user	✓	✓	✓	✓
Imported purchased products for onward sale to UK distributor	✓	✓	✓	–
UK produced purchased products for direct sale to end user	–	–	–	✓
UK produced purchased products for onward sale to distributor	–	–	–	–
Pallets sent to UK end user (new pallets only)	–	–	✓	✓
Pallets sent to UK distributor, who unpacks (new pallets only)	–	–	✓	✓
Products packed for direct sales to UK end user (primary packaging)	–	–	✓	✓
Products packed for sale to UK distributor (primary packaging)	–	–	✓	–
Transit packing to UK direct sales, or to UK distributor who unpacks	–	–	✓	✓
Exports	No obligation (including imported packaging)			
Re-used packaging	No obligation			

Operating Procedure 7:   Issue ......

Dated ..../..../200....

Page: 3 of 5

5. Timescale

The (name) compliance scheme (OR the Environment Agency) requires data to be submitted annually for the preceding calendar year by (date).

6. Sources of data

6.1 Catalogue of packaging weights

A catalogue of packaging weights shall be kept for each product, and updated as more refined data becomes available or when new packaging types or products are introduced.

6.2 Approximations

When approximations have been made, the logic of the approximation must be noted. The Environment Agency has the right to examine data at source and to investigate the realism of approximations.

6.3 Data sources

Data shall be collected from the following sources, in order of preference:

- Direct weighing.
- Data obtained from suppliers.
- By use of the *Ready Reckoner* published by the Department of the Environment, Transport and the Regions 1997.
- By comparison with other similar packaging.

6.4 Bulk purchases of packaging materials

Where packaging materials are bought in bulk, it may be reasonable to assume that packaging despatched is equal to packaging purchased. There will still be a need to divide the total into the sales categories, i.e. direct to UK end user, to UK distributor, to export. It may be acceptable to make this division on the basis of pro-rata invoice values to each category if direct data is not available.

7. Current sources of data

Packaging on imported raw materials	Sample weighings
Strapping on imported raw materials	Sample weighing and estimated metreage
Product and transit packaging on imported products for sale	Suppliers' data
Finished product primary packaging	Unit weights
Finished product transit packaging	Unit weights
Pallets	No. of new pallets purchased at a standard weight
Strapping	Weight purchased. Pro-rated to sales categories

8. Processing the data

The Accountant (OR IT Manager OR . . . . . .) shall arrange for fields to be included in the sales invoicing system to contain packaging weights for each product.

Operating Procedure 7:   Issue . . . . . .

Dated . . . . / . . . . /200 . . . .

Page: 4 of 5

The Environmental Manager (OR . . . . . .) shall set up spreadsheets to collate the quantities and weights, and so derive the data in the format required by the (name) compliance scheme (OR the Environment Agency).

9. Submitting the return

The Environmental Manager (OR . . . . . .) shall prepare the official form, for signature by . . . . . . before being sent to the (name) compliance scheme (OR the Environment Agency).

Operating Procedure 7:   Issue . . . . . .

Dated . . . ./. . . ./200. . . .

Page: 5 of 5

Operating Procedure No. 8

Storage, housekeeping and drainage

1. Purpose and scope

This procedure requires that proper oil/diesel storage facilities are provided, that a good standard of site cleanliness and tidiness is maintained, that a drainage plan is available at all times, and that correct action to prevent pollution is taken in case of spillage.

2. Responsibility

The Engineer (OR Environmental Manager OR . . . . . .) shall be responsible for providing proper oil/diesel storage facilities, for keeping an up-to-date drainage plan and drain marking.

All staff are responsible for maintaining a good standard of housekeeping.

All staff shall immediately deal with spillages to prevent pollution.

The Environmental Manager, or any other Director or Manager, shall be responsible for communicating with the Environment Agency in case of an emergency.

The Engineer (OR . . . . . .) shall be responsible for the maintenance of the interceptor.

3. Oil storage

3.1 Storage tanks

Storage tanks shall either have double skins or be contained within a bund with a capacity not less than 110% of the capacity of the largest tank in the bund. Bunds must be impermeable to water and oil. The whole installation shall be covered to prevent accumulation of rain water.

If there is an accumulation of liquid in the bund, it shall be pumped out and disposed of as special waste.

Bunds shall be inspected at least annually (OR . . . . . .) to prove their integrity.

3.2 Storage in drums and containers

When oil or waste oil is stored in drums or other containers, the drums shall stand within a bund or a drip tray, or stand on stillages over a drip tray. The bund or tray shall have a capacity not less than 25% of the total capacity of containers within the bund/tray.

Spilled oil shall be disposed of as special waste.

Operating Procedure 8:   Issue . . . . . .

Dated . . . ./. . . ./200 . . . .

Page: 1 of 2

3.3 Bowsers

All mobile bowsers shall be fitted with lockable valves which shall be kept locked when not in use.

4. Petroleum storage

The quantity of petroleum spirit which can be held on site is . . . . . . litres as set out in Petroleum Spirit Licence No. . . . . . . issued by . . . . . . Council. The Licence relates to the secure store behind the workshop.

5. Site housekeeping

A high standard of housekeeping, cleanliness and tidiness is required, both to prevent contamination or damage to product or equipment, to prevent accidents and to minimise the risk of pollution.

Sufficient covered skips are provided so that rubbish can be disposed of promptly.

6. Drainage plan

The drainage plan shall be kept up-to-date. A copy shall be on display in the Security Lodge (OR Foreman's Office OR . . . . . .)

Drain covers shall be painted with a coloured arrow to show the direction of flow:

Foul drains   Red
Site drains   Green

7. Spillages

If a spillage of oil or other polluting liquid occurs, the following actions shall be taken:

- Find the source of the spillage and close the valve/tap. If this is not possible, use containers to catch the escaping liquid.
- Impound the escaping liquid so that it cannot enter a surface drain. For large quantities build a sand barrier. For small quantities use the Hazard Response Kit kept in the Security Lodge (OR Foreman's Office OR . . . . . .) or other absorbent medium.

Do not wash the liquid away with water.

- Contaminated absorbents shall be bagged or skipped and disposed of as special waste.

If pollutants enter the site drains and escape from the site, immediately inform the Environmental Manager or other Manager who shall alert the Environment Agency, tel no: (insert telephone number).

8. Interceptor *(if you have one)*

(There will need to be a maintenance regime for skimming and de-sludging any interceptor. The pollutants removed will be special waste. Interceptor maintenance could well be contracted out.)

9. Records

Any spillage which causes pollution or which is potentially polluting shall be recorded on a Nonconformance/Incident Report, noting the circumstances of the incident and the action taken. The Report shall be sent to the Environmental Manager.

```
Operating Procedure 8:   Issue . . . . . .
                    Dated . . . . /. . . . /200. . . .
                                     Page: 2 of 2
```

Operating Procedure No. 9

Maintenance

(Author's note: Maintenance appears as a topic in ISO 9001 under the headings 'process control' (1994) and 'infrastructure' (2000). Maintenance can be even more important in an environmental management system (EMS) particularly if you are required by law to achieve consent conditions. A breakdown of a pump or scrubber, for example, could lead to unacceptable pollution. If you have a planned maintenance system, make sure that your environmental responsibilities are included, e.g. the COSHH Regulations require you to maintain and test LEVs at least every 14 months.)

1. Purpose and scope
This procedure ensures that process, plant and equipment that is essential to keeping control of environmental performance is adequately maintained.

2. Responsibility
The Engineer (OR . . . . . .) is responsible for defining the relevant plant and equipment, scheduling its maintenance and monitoring how the maintenance has been carried out.

The Engineer (OR . . . . . .) shall be satisfied that fitters, electricians, technicians, etc. are competent to carry out the work.

Maintenance staff shall carry out the work and shall record the outcome of the maintenance carried out.

3. Equipment requiring planned maintenance
All equipment which shall be properly operational if the organisation is to satisfy its environmental obligations shall be listed together with the maintenance cycles which must be observed. In determining the maintenance cycles, attention shall be paid to any legislative requirements regarding the frequency of maintenance.

This equipment shall be included in the existing planned maintenance system.

(OR if you do not have a planned maintenance system, write in the following paragraph:)

4. Scheduling maintenance
A schedule shall be maintained showing when each piece of equipment is due for maintenance.

Each week a Work Card shall be prepared for each piece of equipment due for maintenance in the week following.

Work Cards shall be placed ready for maintenance staff or process technicians.)

Operating Procedure 9:   Issue . . . . . .

Dated . . . . / . . . . /200 . . . .

Page: 1 of 2

---

5. Carrying out maintenance

5.1 Competence
Fitters, electricians, technicians, etc. shall be competent to carry out the tasks assigned to them. Their competencies shall be recorded on their Training Records.

5.2 Doing the work
Maintenance staff shall carry out the maintenance as directed. The outcome shall be recorded on the Work Card:

- Description of work done.
- Any additional work identified.
- Any work not completed.
- Signature and date.

6. Follow-up
The Engineer (OR . . . . . .) shall check each completed Work Order. Any uncompleted or additional work shall be scheduled. The Work Card shall be countersigned.

The schedule shall be updated and the Work Order shall be filed under the equipment reference.

(Author's note: This is a manual system. Nowadays such planning and recording is often contained within a computer program.)

Operating Procedure No. 10

Environmental aspects of suppliers and subcontractors

(Author's note: There are many similarities between this procedure and the procedure for approving suppliers and subcontractors in an ISO9001 quality system. It would make sense to add the environmental requirements to the existing quality procedure, but only for those goods and services where there is a perceived environmental impact. The Approved List will need to distinguish between those suppliers and subcontractors who have been granted dual approval, or quality or environment only.)

1. Purpose and scope

This procedure ensures that when the organisation needs to buy goods or services that have a significant environmental aspect, the organisation takes the environmental status of suppliers and subcontractors into account before placing them on the approved list.

2. Responsibility

The Environmental Manager (OR Purchasing Manager OR ......) is responsible for deciding which purchased goods or services have a significant environmental aspect and for evaluating the supplier's or subcontractor's environmental status.

The Environmental Manager (OR ......) is responsible for ensuring that contractors working on site, whether in the long term or short term, have understood and accepted the organisation's environmental responsibilities and procedures.

3. Identifying environmentally sensitive goods and services

The Environmental Manager (OR ......) shall examine the Register of Environmental Aspects to determine which purchased goods or services have a significant environmental aspect. In making this assessment he shall take into account:

- The quantity of the goods or services purchased.
- The resources (raw materials, energy, etc.) that have been consumed in the manufacture of the goods.
- The impact of the supplier's or subcontractor's operations on the environment, under normal, abnormal and emergency conditions.
- Whether the supplier or subcontractor is required to obey any environmental Regulations or Code of Practice.
- If the subcontractor is to work on site, whether there is any risk that through poor management and control of his activities he can cause an environmental incident.

4. Environmental approval of suppliers and subcontractors

4.1 Making enquiries

Having identified the suppliers and subcontractors concerned, the Environmental Manager (OR Purchasing Manager OR . . . . . .) shall send an Environmental Questionnaire (see Annex A) to the supplier or subcontractor for completion and return.

5. Evaluation

An organisation registered to ISO 14001 with an appropriate scope shall be added to the Approved List forthwith. The Environmental Manager (OR . . . . .) shall evaluate the other replies and decide whether to grant approved status. If necessary a visit shall be arranged to view the supplier's or subcontractor's operations or to obtain further information.

Approved suppliers and subcontractors shall be added to the Approved Suppliers List (see Annex B).

6. Contractors working on site

As part of the routine site briefing before contractors start work on site, the Environmental Manager (OR Production Manager OR Engineer OR . . . . . .) shall brief contractors on the environmental risks and responsibilities of the job. Contractors shall nominate a person who shall be responsible for ensuring that the contractor's activities comply with the Operating Procedures, particularly regarding the disposal of wastes and the prevention of pollution. Copies of the relevant Operating Procedures shall be handed to the contractor.

Operating Procedure 10:   Issue . . . . . .

Dated . . . . /. . . . /200. . . .

Page: 2 of 2

(Mr/Mrs/Miss) ....

.... Ltd.

....

....

Dear Mr/Mrs/Miss

Environmental management

(Name of your organisation) is committed to the preservation of the environment and the avoidance of pollution. To improve our control of the environmental aspects of our business we are introducing an environmental management system which meets the requirements of ISO 14001.

It is important to us that our suppliers and subcontractors whose products, services or activities are likely to impact on the environment are themselves likewise concerned about the environment.

We should therefore be pleased if you would complete and return the attached form to us.

If you have any queries or need assistance please contact ....

Yours sincerely

(Job title)

Annex A Oper Proc 10:   Issue ......

Dated ..../..../200....

Page: 1 of 3

ENVIROMENTAL MANAGEMENT
SUPPLIER/SUBCONTRACTOR QUESTIONNAIRE

Name of Company:	
Address:	

Tel No:	Fax No:

Products or services to which this reply applies:

Name of the person who has prime responsibility for environmental performance:

Position:

Are you registered to ISO 14001 or EMAS?	YES/NO

If "yes", state which Standard, and number of the certificate. Please supply a copy showing the scope of your certification.

If ISO 14001, please send us a copy of your Environmental Policy.

If EMAS, please send us a copy of your Environmental Statement.

Then please turn over to sign the form, and return it to us.

Annex A Oper Proc 10: Issue . . . . . .

Dated . . . . /. . . . /200. . . .

Page: 2 of 3

If you are *not* certified, please answer the following questions:	
Do you have an Environmental Management System?	
Do you have an Environmental Policy? If "yes", please send us a copy.	YES/NO
Are you currently preparing for ISO 14001 or EMAS?	YES/NO
If "yes", when do you expect to be approved?	
If "no":	
Have you defined the environmental Regulations which apply to your organisation?	YES/NO
Have you defined the environmental impacts caused by your activities?	YES/NO
Are there written procedures to control environmental activities, especially emergencies?	YES/NO
Do you measure environmental performance?	YES/NO
Is environmental performance regularly reviewed by senior management?	YES/NO
Do your training plans include environmental training?	YES/NO
Please send us a copy of your statment of environmental impacts, if available	ENCLOSED/ NOT AVAILABLE
Please send us a copy of your list of relevant environmental Regulations, if available.	ENCLOSED/ NOT AVAILABLE
Have you given consideration to the environmental impact associated with the production of your purchased raw materials, components, etc., and the ultimate disposal of your product?	YES/NO

Signed: ....

Position in Company: ....

Date: ....

Please return to:

Annex A Oper Proc 10:   Issue ...... Dated ..../..../200.... Page: 3 of 3

APPROVED SUPPLIERS LIST

Supplier/Subcontractor Details	Scope of goods/services provided	Basis of Approval e.g. ISO 14001, Questionnaire, Visit, etc.	Comments

Annex B Oper Proc 10: Issue . . . .

Dated . . . ./. . . ./200 . . . . .

Page: 1 of 1

Operating Procedure No. 11

Energy control and monitoring

1. Purpose and scope

This procedure describes the actions to be taken to reduce energy (gas and electricity) consumption, which is one of the organisation's environmental improvement objectives.

This procedure sets out how energy consumption shall be controlled and monitored.

2. Responsibility

All staff are responsible for conserving electricity and heat.

The Electrician (OR Engineer OR . . . . . .) is responsible for the ongoing programme of introducing sensors and other energy saving devices, and for programming the 7-day clock.

The Engineer (OR . . . . . .) is responsible for checking for compressed air leaks.

The Electrician (OR Engineer OR Environmental Manager OR . . . . . .) is responsible for meter readings.

The Environmental Manager (OR . . . . . .) is responsible for analysing the consumption figures and initiating any necessary corrective action.

3. Control of electricity usage

All lights shall be turned off when daylight is sufficient or the room, etc. is not in use.

There is an on-going programme to install sensors in common areas, e.g. reception, corridors, toilets.

All computers shall be programmed to power down/power off VDUs when the computer is idle.

There shall be weekly checks for leaks in the compressed air system. Leaks shall be mended. The compressor shall be turned off one hour before the end of the working day; the receiver holds sufficient air for operations to continue.

4. Control of heating

All central heating radiators are thermostatically controlled. If an area becomes too hot, reduce the thermostat before opening windows. All windows shall be closed when a room is vacated.

Operating Procedure 11:   Issue . . . . . .

Dated . . . ./. . . ./200. . . .

Page: 1 of 2

Doors into the factory and warehouse shall be kept shut when not in use. Doors with high levels of traffic will be fitted with automatic opening doors or air curtains in due course.

The 7-day control clock shall be reset each week to conform to the working pattern in the next seven days.

5. Energy monitoring

5.1 Meter reading

The gas company's, electricity company's and the company's own submeters shall be read on the first Monday of every month.

Meters are located at:

Gas company	Meter house (yard)
Electricity company	Sub-station
Office sub-meter	Switch room
Factory sub-meter	Switch room

The readings shall be entered on the clipboard sheet kept in each location.

5.2 Analysis

The readings and the number of working weeks that have elapsed since the previous reading shall be entered into the computer spreadsheet.

The consumption for each location (in kWh per working week and kWh per unit of production OR other appropriate measurement) shall be plotted on the annual graph and compared with the previous year and with the planned consumption for the current year.

Any significant deviations from plan shall be investigated, and the findings discussed with the managers or staff responsible for the department or area. Corrective action shall be taken.

5.3 Reporting

Progress, findings and a report on any corrective action taken shall be reported to the environmental management review meeting.

(Author's note: You should take your own meter readings at the time you choose. It is no good relying on the gas or electricity company's invoices. They read meters at irregular intervals and often estimate consumption. Installing submeters to measure local electricity consumptions often gives worthwhile data which points to where savings can be made.)

Operating Procedure No. 12

Company cars

1. Purpose and scope
This procedure ensures that the administration of the car fleet, the selection of cars and driving skills are carried out in a way which will minimise environmental impact.

2. Responsibility
The Company Secretary (OR Administrator OR . . . . . .) is responsible for the operation of the company's car fleet, and for monitoring environmental performance.

All drivers shall drive with due attention to fuel economy and tyre wear.

3. Selection of cars
When a new car is to be purchased, the Company Secretary (OR Administrator OR . . . . . .) shall select cars taking into account the emissions indices published by the Department of the Environment, Transport and the Regions (OR When a company driver is to have a new car, the Company Secretary (OR Administrator OR . . . . . .) shall ensure that the driver is aware of the data on emissions indices and the effect these will have on the taxable car benefit).

4. Driving skills
The company shall arrange for every company driver to attend a driving skills course, with particular emphasis on defensive driving, fuel economy and preserving tyre life.

5. Records
All drivers shall keep a record of the quantity of fuel purchased and mileage travelled, and of tyres purchased and mileage travelled.

These figures shall be given to the Company Secretary (OR Administrator OR . . . . . .) every . . . . . . months, to be entered into the computer spreadsheet to calculate consumptions.

Where a driver shows an abnormal level of miles per litre, or of miles per tyre, the situation shall be investigated.

Operating Procedure No. 13

Environmental objectives and targets

(Author's note: This procedure is written using the convention that all environmental impacts are detrimental. The introduction to the model Register of Environmental Aspects discusses the possibility of beneficial impacts. If you want to use this concept, then the table set out in the introduction should be substituted into this procedure.)

1. Purpose and scope

This procedure sets out how the organisation shall determine the relative significance of environmental aspects, set objectives and targets for improvement, and set the resulting action plans and progress them to completion.

2. Responsibility

The Environmental Manager is responsible for ranking the significance of environmental aspects, presenting the results to the environmental management meeting, writing and circulating environmental action plans, progressing the plans and reporting to management.

The environmental management review meeting sets improvement plans.

Designated people manage improvement plans to completion.

3. Determining the significance of an environmental aspect

3.1 Definitions

Normal   This includes all normal operations occurring on site.

Abnormal   This includes reasonably foreseeable situations that do not involve the emergency services.

Emergency   This includes any incident that does or could involve the emergency services.

Each aspect defined in the Register of Environmental Aspects shall be rated against each definition. Note that all the definitions may not always apply, e.g. some aspects may never create abnormal or emergency conditions; other aspects may only come into play if there is an emergency.

Operating Procedure 13:   Issue . . . . . .

Dated . . . . / . . . . /200 . . . .

Page: 1 of 3

3.2 Relative significance of environmental aspects

The relative impact shall be calculated using the following equation:

Impact = Frequency of occurrence × Severity using the following scale:

Frequency of occurrence		Severity	
Description	Factor	Description	Factor
Unlikely (less than once a year)	1	Minimal environmental impact	1
Common (monthly/several times a year)	2	Low environmental impact	2
Frequent (daily/weekly)	3	Moderate environmental impact	3
		High environmental impact	6
		Severe environmental impact	10

'Severity' shall take into account the following:

- The scale of the operation (e.g. although car emissions on a national scale have a severe environmental impact, your severity will be low if you only have two company cars).
- If prosecution because of failing to observe the law will have an adverse effect on the organisation's finances or reputation, a higher severity rating may be justified than that which would be related to the environmental impact on its own.

3.3 Ranking significance

The Environmental Manager shall prepare a significance table to rank the aspects and their significance, using the 'Significance of environmental aspects' form (see Annex A).

3.4 Review

The Register of Environmental Aspects and the significance of aspects shall be reviewed and updated at least annually, and also if there is any significant change to processes, equipment or operational practices. Note shall be taken of any incidents, complaints or audit findings.

Operating Procedure 13:   Issue . . . . . .

Dated . . . . / . . . . /200 . . . .

Page: 2 of 3

4. Setting improvement objectives and targets

4.1 Management review

The environmental management review meeting shall use the significance table to select which aspects shall be included in the environmental improvement programme and which shall be subject to formal Operating Procedures.

As a guide, aspects showing a significance of 6 or more shall always be reviewed. Aspects with a significance less than 6 shall be actioned as the opportunity arises.

The objective and target setting activity shall also take into account:

- The Environmental Policy.
- Legislation.
- The views of any interested parties.
- The need to prevent pollution in general.

4.2 Environmental improvement plans

Each objective or target shall be set out on an Environmental Action Plan (see Annex B) which shall state:

- The objective or target.
- The stages of the project.
- The timetable.
- Who is responsible for managing the project.

Environmental Action Plans shall be circulated to the people concerned.

5. Progressing and review of improvement plans

The progress of improvement shall be monitored and recorded on the Environmental Action Plan.

Progress to date shall be reported at each environmental management review meeting. Plans shall be updated or revised as decided by the meeting.

SIGNIFICANCE OF ENVIRONMENTAL ASPECTS

Aspect	Impact – normal	Impact – abnormal	Impact – emergency	Comment/action

Compiled by: ....

Date: ....

ENVIRONMENTAL ACTION PLAN

TITLE:

OBJECTIVE:

Adopted at Management Meeting held on:

PLAN

Action	Action by	Start date	Completion date	Date completed

Progress/revision dates (see over)				

Annex B Oper Proc 13:   Issue . . . . . .

Dated . . . . / . . . . /200 . . . .

Page: 1 of 2

186

PROGRESS NOTES

Date	Progress notes	Initials

Annex B Oper Proc 13:   Issue . . . . . .

Dated . . . ./ . . . ./200 . . . .

Page: 2 of 2

Operating Procedure No. 14

New products and processes

1. Purpose and scope

This procedure ensures that the environmental implications of new products and new or changed processes, plant and equipment are taken into account when the decision to proceed is being taken, along with such considerations as finance, profitability, markets, health and safety.

This procedure embraces aspects of life cycle assessment.

2. Responsibility

The Directors are responsible for ensuring that environmental factors are taken into account when new developments are being planned.

3. New products

When designing new products, the environmental aspects associated with the product's manufacture and eventual use shall be taken into account, e.g.:

3.1 Choice of raw materials

The environmental impacts associated with the production of the selected raw materials, e.g. resources, energy, pollution, transport, etc.

3.2 Manufacturing

- Process yields, i.e. waste minimisation.
- Energy usage.
- Water usage.
- Wastes likely to be generated and their disposal.
- Emissions.
- Effluents.
- Prescribed processes under the *Environmental Protection Act 1990*.
- Design and minimisation of packaging – *Packaging (Essential Requirements) Regulations 1998*.
- etc.

3.3 In use

- Product life.
- Energy efficiency.
- Water consumption.
- etc.

3.4 Ultimate disposal
- Ease of recycling.

4. New, or changes to, processes and plant development
When planning new, or changes to, processes, plant or equipment, the environmental aspects of the process or the equipment shall be taken into account, e.g.:

4.1 Manufacture
- Resources, energy, etc., used in its manufacture.

4.2 In operation
- Energy efficiency.
- Water consumption.
- Emissions.
- Effluents.
- Prescribed processes under the *Environmental Protection Act 1990*.
- Planning requirements.
- Risk of an emergency.

4.3 When redundant
- How will the plant or equipment be disposed of?

Operating Procedure 14:   Issue . . . . . .

Dated . . . . / . . . . /200 . . . .

Page: 2 of 2

Operating Procedure No. 15

Environmental training

(Author's note: This procedure parallels the requirements for training in ISO 9001, except for the added requirements that staff should know the environmental implications of departing from the set procedures. However, this same requirement in respect of quality is now included in ISO9001:2000. It would make sense to revise any existing quality system procedure, call it 'Training' and expand the scope to include both quality and environment, rather than write and maintain a separate environmental procedure.)

1. Purpose and scope
This procedure ensures that all staff receive environmental awareness training, and specific training in the environmental responsibilities and likely environmental impact of their individual jobs, and that training records are kept.

2. Responsibility
The Managing Director (OR Personnel Manager OR Departmental Manager OR ......) ensures that all staff and new starters receive environmental awareness training.

Departmental Managers (OR Supervisors OR ......) ensure that all staff receive specific training in the environmental implications and responsibilities of their job.

The Training Department (OR ......) keeps and maintains training records.

3. Environmental awareness training
All staff shall receive training in environmental awareness including the major environmental impacts of the organisation's activities and the Environmental Policy and be introduced to the environmental management system and its Operating Procedures.

Awareness training shall be a part of the induction training for all new starters at any level in the organisation. This shall include temporary staff.

4. Job training
All staff shall be trained in the specific environmental impacts, actual or potential, and the environmental responsibilities associated with their job, and the relevant procedures including emergency procedures. They shall understand the potential consequences of departing from the specified procedures.

5. Competence and training needs
The competence and training needs of each member of staff shall be reviewed regularly, at least annually. Any training identified shall be provided, whether in-house or externally.

Operating Procedure 15: Issue ......

Dated ..../..../200....

Page: 1 of 2

6. Training records

There shall be a Training Record (see Annex A) for each employee, including Directors, which shall show when reviews have been carried out, training needs identified and training given.

Evidence of formal training, e.g. certificates of courses attended, shall be attached to an individual's record.

TRAINING RECORD

NAME: JOB TITLE:

DATE STARTED WITH COMPANY:

Details of qualification/experience	Date obtained	Verified

Recommended training	Date planned	Date received	Employee's signature to confirm training received	Comments
Induction				
Safety awareness				
Quality awareness				
Envtl awareness				

Annex A Oper Proc 15:   Issue ......

Dated ..../..../200....

Page: 1 of 1

Operating Procedure No. 16

Environmental communications

1. Purpose and scope

This procedure ensures that all communications received by the organisation from external parties relating to its environmental performance are properly handled.

The procedure also addresses the requirements for communication within the organisation relating to the environment.

2. Responsibility

Any member of staff receiving complaints or communications from external parties shall pass them to the appropriate person for investigation and action.

The Environmental Manager has the main responsibility for responding to requests, but shall seek advice if necessary.

The Environmental Manager is responsible for circulating environmental information within the organisation.

3. External complaints

Any member of staff receiving a complaint about environmental performance from an external source shall direct the complainant to the Environmental Manager, or if the Environmental Manager is not available, to (name).

The details of the complaint shall be entered on a Nonconformance/Incident Report:

- Complainant's name, address and telephone number.
- Details of the complaint.
- Day and time the problem occurred.

The complaint shall be explored in sufficient detail for the likely source of the problem to be identified.

The Environmental Manager shall investigate the complaint; this shall include consideration as to whether the incident is likely to create an environmental hazard.

The complaint shall be followed up as set out in Operating Procedure 19 'Nonconformance, corrective and preventive action'.

The Environmental Manager (OR . . . . . .) shall respond to the complainant.

4. Requests for information

Requests for information, either from trading partners, e.g. customers, or the general public, shall be directed to the Environmental Manager. The Environmental Manager shall confer with the Managing Director (OR . . . . . .) if there is any doubt about how to reply, e.g. the matter may be confidential. The Environmental Manager shall respond to the enquirer.

If appropriate, the Environmental Manager is authorised to release an 'uncontrolled' copy of the Environmental Policy or the Environmental Management Manual.

Note that the Environmental Policy shall be freely available to the public and other interested parties on request.

5. Communication with the regulators

The Environmental Manager (OR . . . . . .) shall be the organisation's representative in all dealings with the regulators, e.g. Environmental Agency, local authority.

6. Internal communications

The requirements of the environmental management system are communicated to all staff through:

- Training (see Operating Procedure 15 'Environmental training').
- The distribution of Operating Procedures and Work Instructions (see Operating Procedure 17 'Document control').

Any defects found in the operation of the environmental management system requiring immediate attention shall be circulated by memo.

Operating Procedure 16:   Issue . . . . . .

Dated . . . . / . . . . /200 . . . .

Page: 2 of 2

Operating Procedure No. 17

Document control

(Author's note: This procedure parallels the requirements for document control in ISO 9001. It would make sense to add the environmental requirements, including the section on environmental legislation, to any existing quality system procedure and to expand the scope to include both quality and environment, rather than writing and maintaining a separate environmental procedure.)

1. Purpose and scope
This procedure sets out how the documents required to run the environmental management system (EMS) are created, authorised, distributed, revised and updated.

2. Responsibility
The Environmental Manager (OR . . . . . .) is responsible for the administration of document control procedures, obtaining the correct authorisations, maintaining document identity and issue status, controlling distribution, updating, and keeping archive files.

3. Controlled documents

3.1 Definition
'Controlled documents' are documents which must be authorised before issue, are given an issue and/or revision status and are issued to named recipients who are automatically sent revisions and re-issues and who acknowledge receipt of the document.

The controlled documents in this EMS are:

- Environmental Management Manual.
- Register of Environmental Aspects.
- Register of Environmental Legislation.
- Operating Procedures.
- (Work Instructions).

3.2 Authorisation
Each issue or revision of a controlled document shall be authorised by the appropriate person:

- Environmental Management Manual   Managing Director
- Registers   Managing Director (OR . . . . . .)
- Operating Procedures   Managing Director (OR . . . . . .)
- (Work Instructions)   Managing Director (OR . . . . . .)

The authorisation shall be recorded on the document, or on an Authorisation and Amendment Control Sheet (see Annex A) held by the Environmental Manager.

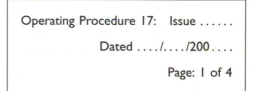

Operating Procedure 17:   Issue . . . . . .

Dated . . . . ./. . . . ./200 . . . .

Page: 1 of 4

3.3 Page layout
All documents shall display a page count, e.g. page 1 of 6.

3.4 Issue and revision status
All documents shall carry the date they were created.

The Manual and the Registers, being large documents, shall carry an issue number and a revision number. If only individual pages are revised, the revision number of those pages shall be raised by one, the issue number staying the same. If the whole document is re-issued, the issue number shall be raised by one and the revision number returned to zero.

Operating Procedures and Work Instructions should ideally carry an issue number, but this is not compulsory; they can be controlled on date alone. When any part of one of these documents is revised, the whole document shall be re-issued.

The Authorisation and Amendment Control Sheet shall be used to keep a record of the details of issues (and revisions) for each document.

3.5 Identification of changes
Text which has been changed shall be identified by highlighting, change of font, margin marks, etc. The identification shall be restored to normal before further revisions are made.

3.6 Distribution
The organisation may only need one copy of some documents, e.g. the Manual and the Registers. The master copy shall be held by the Environmental Manager (OR . . . . . .).

When distribution is needed, the List of Copy Holders (see Annex B) shall be used to show which people should hold a copy. The initials of each recipient shall be obtained on the List to confirm receipt. (If necessary, distribution can be made under cover of a memo which shall be signed and returned to confirm receipt.)

3.7 Archives
When documents are re-issued or revised, a copy of the original document or pages shall be placed in an archive file.

3.8 Documents held on computer for direct reference
Where documents are held on computer for direct reference there is no need for formal records of issues and distribution. The document shall carry a record showing the date created or last amended.

The document shall carry the identity of the person who is allowed to change the text, and the name of the person who has authorised it for distribution.

When any such document is altered, the pages that have been changed shall be printed off, be correctly authorised and placed in date order in an archive file. Staff shall be advised, e.g. by e-mail, that an alteration has been made.

Operating Procedure 17:   Issue . . . . . .

Dated . . . . /. . . . /200 . . . .

Page: 2 of 4

If any computer-held document is printed for any purpose, the printed copy shall be 'uncontrolled' and shall be destroyed after use.

3.9 Uncontrolled documents

If a copy of a controlled document is issued for information only, e.g. to a customer, it shall be marked 'confidential' and 'uncontrolled'. A record shall be kept of its issue but it shall not be included in any re-issue or revision process.

4. Forms

A copy of the current version of each form shall be kept in a master file. The file shall be indexed (see Annex C).

Issue status shall be denoted by the date the form was created. The date of the current version shall be noted in the index.

5. Documents of external origin

5.1 Master copies

The Environmental Manager shall keep the master copy of all reference documents of external origin, e.g. British Standards, copies of legislation, codes of practice.

5.2 Updating ISO 14001 and other standards

The certification body (name) will inform the organisation of any changes to ISO 14001 (OR The organisation is a member of BSI and receives *BSI News* which gives details of new and revised Standards OR The organisation subscribes to the BSI Plus service and will automatically be informed of any changes to the Standard OR The organisation has made an arrangement with its consultants that they will inform the organisation of any changes to the Standard(s) OR There shall be an annual check that the Standard(s) has not been changed, e.g. by telephoning BSI; each copy shall be marked 'still current' with initials and date.)

5.3 Updating legislation

There shall be a means of ensuring that the organisation is kept up-to-date with any changes to environmental legislation, codes of practice, etc. that are relevant.

This shall be done through membership of the (name) Trade Association (OR by subscribing to an up-date service, e.g. Tolley's Environmental Law and Procedures Management OR other reference documents which are regularly updated OR by retaining the services of a consultant to review environmental legislation and report regularly to the Environmental Manager).

The Environmental Manager shall incorporate any changes to existing legislation, or any new relevant legislation, into the Register of Legislation.

5.4 Obtaining up-to-date documents

When a document of external origin is found to have been updated, the Environmental Manager (OR . . . . . .) shall decide whether there is a need to obtain a new copy immediately or not.

Operating Procedure 17: Issue . . . . . .

Dated . . . . / . . . . /200 . . . .

Page: 3 of 4

In either case, the existing copy shall be marked 'uncontrolled' until a new copy is obtained. Documents marked 'uncontrolled' shall be used for information only; if the document is required for definitive use, the user shall check that the relevant text is still current; if not, an up-to-date copy shall be obtained.

6. Obsolete documents

When documents are revised, they shall be issued to all locations where they are needed for the efficient functioning of the environmental management system and obsolete documents shall be withdrawn.

Where obsolete or invalid documents need to be retained for legal or historical reasons, they shall clearly be marked as withdrawn.

7. Legibility

Every person who fills in a form or other record shall ensure that everything, including any initials or signature, is legible.

8. Retention times

Retention times and computer back-up procedures are defined in Operating Procedure 20 'Environmental records'.

Operating Procedure 17:   Issue . . . . . .

Dated . . . . / . . . . /200 . . . .

Page: 4 of 4

DOCUMENT TITLE:	

AUTHORISATION AND AMENDMENT
CONTROL SHEET

Date	Issue no.	Revn no.	Page no.	Modification	Authorised by

Annex A Oper Proc 17:   Issue . . . . . .

Dated . . . . / . . . . /200 . . . .

Page: 1 of 1

DOCUMENT TITLE:	

LIST OF CONTROLLED COPY HOLDERS

		Issue/revision date:				
Copy no.	Pages	Holder	Holder's initials			

Annex B Oper Proc 17: Issue . . . . . .

Dated . . . . / . . . . /200 . . . .

Page: 1 of 1

INDEX OF FORMS

Document	Ref. no.	Date	Date	Date	Date

Annex C Oper Proc 17: Issue . . . . . .

Dated . . . ./. . . ./200. . . .

Page: 1 of 1

Operating Procedure No. 18

Monitoring and measuring equipment

(Author's note: This procedure parallels the requirements for control of inspection, measuring and test equipment in ISO 9001. It would make sense to add any measuring and control equipment involved in the environmental system which requires calibration to the list of equipment in the quality system and to expand the scope to include both quality and environment, rather than writing and maintaining a separate environmental procedure.

Examples of equipment which would be required to implement some of the model Operating Procedures are: weighbridges, weighing scales and load cells; electricity, gas and water meters; pH meters; chemical analytical equipment; sampling equipment; thermocouples and temperature alarms; plant operational failure alarms.)

1. Purpose and scope
This procedure ensures that equipment used to measure, monitor or control environmental operating parameters is maintained and calibrated to preserve its efficiency and accuracy.

2. Responsibility
The Environmental Manager (OR Engineer OR . . . . . .) is responsible for defining measuring and monitoring equipment which needs to be maintained or calibrated and ensuring that action is taken at the correct time. The results of calibration are assessed and appropriate action taken if equipment has fallen out of calibration. Records are kept.

3. Equipment to be calibrated or maintained
Each piece of equipment that requires calibration or regular maintenance shall be uniquely identified. Ideally, identification shall use the serial number or an index number etched on the piece of equipment, or if this is not feasible, by indelible labelling.

4. Calibration

4.1 Records
Each piece of equipment shall have a Calibration/Maintenance Record (see Annex A), which shall set out:

- Frequency of calibration.
- Method of calibration.
- Allowable tolerances.
- Dates calibration carried out.

Operating Procedure 18:   Issue . . . . . .

Dated . . . . / . . . . /200 . . . .

Page: 1 of 2

- Actual readings obtained.
- Comments on the acceptability of the results.
- Any subsequent action taken.

4.2 Methods of calibration

Unless the equipment is marked 'For indication purposes only' all calibrations shall be traceable to nationally recognised standards. If this is not possible, the basis of the method of calibration shall be stated.

When appropriate or necessary, an approved external calibration service may be used. This can be the original manufacturer or his agent, or a NAMAS or ISO 9001 approved test house.

Calibration shall be carried out in suitable working environment conditions.

4.3 Results of calibration

The results of calibration shall be compared with the tolerance. When calibration is carried out by a subcontractor, the results shall be reviewed and, if acceptable, the certificate shall be initialled and dated. If calibration is satisfactory, the Calibration/Maintenance Record shall be marked 'OK'.

5. Calibration failure

If a piece of equipment falls out of tolerance, it shall be withdrawn from use and repaired and re-calibrated, or be withdrawn permanently and replaced.

The validity of measurements taken prior to the failure shall be reviewed and a decision taken whether any retrospective action needs to be taken.

6. Retest dates

Ideally, when equipment has been calibrated it should be labelled to show the next retest date. Retest dates shall also be shown on a schedule (see Annex B) or be part of a computer based recall program.

7. Test software

Software used for measuring and monitoring shall be validated prior to use.

Operating Procedure 18:   Issue ......

Dated ..../..../200....

Page: 2 of 2

CALIBRATION/MAINTENANCE RECORD

Serial no/identity	
Description	
Location	
Calibration method	
Frequency	

Check readings at			
Allowed tolerance			

Date	Reading 1	Reading 2	Reading 3	Comment

Annex A Oper Proc 18:   Issue ......

Dated ..../..../200....

Page: 1 of 1

SCHEDULE OF EQUIPMENT TO BE
CALIBRATED/MAINTAINED
YEAR 200....

Identity	Description	Location	Jan	Feb	Mar	Apr	May	Jun	Jly	Aug	Sep	Oct	Nov	Dec

Annex B Oper Proc 18:   Issue ......

Dated ..../..../200....

Page: 1 of 1

Operating Procedure No. 19

Nonconformance, corrective and preventive action

1. Purpose and scope

This procedure ensures that if and when an environmental incident occurs or an environmental complaint is received, the circumstances are investigated and appropriate short-term corrective action and longer-term preventive action is taken and followed up.

2. Responsibility

All staff are responsible for reporting environmental incidents.

The Environmental Manager in conjunction with other managers agrees what preventive action is required and ensures that the action is taken and is effective.

The Environmental Manager reports on incidents to management.

3. Environmental incidents

Environmental incidents may arise from:

- A failure to observe Operating Procedures.
- An inadequate Operating Procedure.
- Unforeseen circumstances, e.g. abnormal operating conditions.
- Emergencies.
- Complaints.

4. Registering the incident

Any person who becomes aware of an incident shall record the details on an Environmental Nonconformance/Incident Report (see Annex A), and shall fill in the following details:

- Origin or location of the incident.
- A description of the incident.
- Any immediate corrective action taken to overcome or contain the incident.
- If appropriate, make proposals for long-term preventive action which will prevent a repeat of the incident or similar incidents. These proposals may require a revision to an existing Operating Procedure, or the writing of a new procedure.

The form shall be sent to the Environmental Manager.

Operating Procedure 19:   Issue ......

Dated ..... / ..... /200 ....

Page: 1 of 2

5. Preventive action

The Environmental Manager shall discuss the incident with the Managing Director (OR Departmental Manager OR Supervisor concerned) and shall agree whether any long-term preventive action is appropriate or not. The details shall be entered on the Report form, and shall be circulated to the relevant people.

6. Follow-up

The Environmental Manager shall in due course check that the preventive action has been completed and that it has been effective, or is likely to be effective, in preventing a repeat of the incident. The form shall then be signed off.

7. Reporting to management

The Environmental Manager shall prepare a brief report summarising the incidents, their impact and the resulting action taken and submit it to the environmental management review meeting for discussion.

Operating Procedure 19:   Issue . . . . . .

Dated . . . . /. . . . /200 . . . .

Page: 2 of 2

ENVIRONMENTAL
NONCONFORMANCE/INCIDENT REPORT

External contact (if relevant):	Date:	Report no.
Department/site:	Raised by:	

Description of incident/nonconformance:

Short-term action taken:

Action taken by: Date:

Proposed long-term preventive action:

Proposed by: Date:

Action to be taken:	Action to be taken by:
	Date by:
	Action taken:
	Date:

Form to be sent to the Environment Manager when completed

Verified as effective:	Date:

Annex A Oper Proc 19:   Issue . . . . . .

Dated . . . . / . . . . /200 . . . .

Page: 1 of 1

Operating Procedure No. 20

Environmental records

(Author's note: This procedure parallels the requirements for control of quality records in ISO 9001. If you have a quality management system, then expand its scope to include both quality and environment and add the titles of your environment records to the list of documents with their location, retention times, etc.

Make sure that any documents required by law are retained for the statutory length of time.)

1. Purpose and scope

This procedure ensures that all documents and records that form part of the environmental management system are stored securely and have a stipulated retention time. In some cases the retention time is required by statute. The procedure also sets out the back-up routine for documents held on computer.

2. Responsibility

The Environmental Manager plays the major part in the retention of environmental records, but other members of staff are designated to hold certain records as detailed in this procedure.

3. Documents to be retained

The documents that are to be retained, their location and the retention times are listed in the following table.

The three year retention period for documents that demonstrate the performance of the environmental management system is in accord with the three year review cycle set by UKAS.

Remember that when statutory documents have an extended period of validity (e.g. annual Transfer Notes), the retention time starts when the document expires.

All records are to be identified, collated, indexed, filed, and stored securely so that they will not deteriorate and can be retrieved straightforwardly if required.

Records may be disposed of on the authority of the holder when the retention time has expired.

4. Computer records

Computer records shall be backed up every day (OR week OR computer transactions shall be backed up daily and the files backed up monthly). Alternate sets of back-up tapes (OR disks) shall be used. The current set of tapes (OR disks) shall be kept in a fireproof safe (OR securely off site). Periodic tests shall be made to ensure that back-ups can be read and are not corrupted.

Operating Procedure 20: Issue . . . . . .

Dated . . . . / . . . . / 200 . . . .

Page: 1 of 4

Document	Raised by	Retained by	Retention time (years)
Environmental Management Manual	Environmental Manager	Environmental Manager	3
Register of Environmental Aspects	Environmental Manager	Environmental Manager	3
Register of Environmental Legislation	Environmental Manager	Environmental Manager	3
Operating Procedures	Environmental Manager	Environmental Manager	3
Work Instructions	Environmental Manager	Environmental Manager	3
Controlled Waste Transfer Notes	Person handing over waste	Environmental Manager	2
Special Waste Consignment Notes	Person handing over waste	Environmental Manager	3
Waste Carrier Licences	Environmental Agency	Environmental Manager	Period of validity + 1
Approved Contractors & Suppliers	Environmental Manager	Environmental Manager	3
Energy monitoring records	Environmental Manager (OR . . . .)	Environmental Manager	3
Water monitoring records	Environmental Manager (OR . . . .)	Environmental Manager	3
Local authority/Environment Agency licences	Local authority/ Environment Agency	Environmental Manager (OR Company Secretary)	Period of validity + 1

Operating Procedure 20: Issue . . . .

Dated . . . . / . . . . /200 . . . . .

Page: 2 of 4

210

Document	Raised by	Retained by	Retention time (years)
Environmental communications from external sources	External	Environmental Manager	3
Environmental Action Plans	Environmental Manager	Environmental Manager	3
Packaging data	Environmental Manager	Environmental Manager	3
Audit schedules	Environmental Manager	Environmental Manager	3
Audit reports	Auditor	Environmental Manager	3
Assessment reports	Certification body	Environmental Manager	3
Corrective/Preventive Action Form	Environmental Manager	Environmental Manager	3
Training Records	Personnel (OR Manager)	Personnel (OR Manager)	Period of employment + 1
Environmental Nonconformance/Incident Report	Any member of staff	Environmental Manager	3
Management Review minutes	Environmental Manager	Environmental Manager	3
Water treatment log sheets	Operator	Technical Manager	3
Solvent Register	Paint Technician	Paint Store and then Environmental Manager	3

Document	Raised by	Retained by	Retention time (years)
Solvent Odour Book	Security	Security Office and then Environmental Manager	3
Authorisation and Amendment Control Sheet	Environmental Manager	Environmental Manager	3
List of Copy Holders	Environmental Manager	Environmental Manager	3
Index of Forms	Environmental Manager	Environmental Manager	3
Copies of Standards	BSI etc	Environmental Manager	Period of validity + 1
Copies of legislation, codes of practice	External agencies	Environmental Manager	Period of validity + 1
Schedule of equipment to be calibrated/maintained	Environmental Manager (OR Engineer)	Environmental Manager (OR Engineer)	3
Calibration/Maintenance Record	Environmental Manager (OR Engineer)	Environmental Manager (OR Engineer)	3
Calibration certificates	External test house	Environmental Manager (OR Engineer)	3
Maintenance Work Cards	Engineer	Engineer	1

Operating Procedure 20: Issue ....
Dated ..... / ..... /200 .....
Page: 4 of 4

Operating Procedure No. 21

Internal environmental audits

(Author's note: This procedure parallels the requirements for internal auditing in ISO 9001. It would make sense to add the environmental requirements to any existing quality system procedure, calling it 'Internal Audits', rather then writing and maintaining a separate environmental procedure.)

1. Purpose and scope

This procedure ensures that effective internal environmental audits are carried out as a means of maintaining the effectiveness of the environmental management system (EMS).

2. Responsibility

The Managing Director (OR . . . . . .) decides who is to be appointed as environmental auditors. Whilst ideally auditors should be members of the organisation, some or all of the audits may be subcontracted to a suitably qualified and experienced subcontract person or consultancy.

The Environmental Manager ensures that auditors are trained and are competent, draws up the audit schedule, progresses corrective and preventive actions found to be necessary as a result of an audit, and reports to the environmental management review meeting.

Auditors carry out audits in a comprehensive and responsible manner, and prepare audit findings reports for discussion with local management and the Environmental Manager.

3. Auditors

Auditors shall have received training in the responsibilities and skills of internal environmental auditing.

Auditors shall be managerially independent of the activity being audited.

Auditors shall be alert to the environmental impact of the activities they are auditing and shall draw the attention of the Environmental Manager to any aspect which they feel is not adequately represented in the EMS.

4. Audit schedule

The Environmental Manager shall prepare a list of environmental audit topics (see Annex A) so that all parts of the EMS are allocated to a topic.

At the start of each year, the Environmental Manager shall prepare an Audit Schedule (see Annex B) which shall show the topics for audit and the frequency of audits. The frequency

Operating Procedure 21:   Issue . . . . . .

Dated . . . . / . . . . /200 . . . .

Page: 1 of 3

of audits shall be based on the importance of the topic and the outcome of previous audits.

Every topic shall be audited at least once a year. Repeat audits shall be scheduled at any time if an audit shows significant shortcomings that need to be corrected quickly. Audits shall be carried out within one month either side of the scheduled month.

5. The audit

Auditors shall first review the outcome of any previous audit of the topic and check that there are no outstanding corrective or preventive actions.

Auditors shall plan the audit using information from the relevant clauses of the Environmental Management Manual, the relevant Operating Procedures (and any associated Work Instructions).

Auditors shall seek evidence to test the requirements of the environmental management system are being fulfilled.

6. Audit report

Auditors shall record in the Audit Report (see Annex B) the reference to the part of the EMS which has been audited, the evidence examined and the outcome.

Findings shall be categorised:

OK   where the finding is satisfactory.
NC   where there is a noncompliance with the requirements of the EMS.
OBS   where a weakness is found which if not addressed could lead to a future noncompliance.
IMPR   where proposals are made which would improve the effectiveness of the EMS or the organisation's performance.

Auditors shall make recommendations for corrective and preventive action if possible. Auditors shall present the Audit Report to the Environmental Manager who shall draw it to the attention of the person concerned.

7. Short-term corrective action

The Environmental Manager shall ensure that any short-term corrective actions are carried out promptly and sign them off on the Report.

8. Long-term corrective and preventive actions

Long-term corrective and preventive actions shall be agreed with the relevant directors, managers or supervisors.

The agreed actions shall be written into a Corrective/Preventive Action Form (see Annex C) which shall be sent to the person responsible for taking action.

If the audit finding indicates a weakness or mistake within the EMS, the Operating Procedures shall be changed to correct the situation.

Operating Procedure 21:   Issue . . . . . .

Dated . . . . /. . . . /200 . . . .

Page: 2 of 3

9. Follow-up

The Environmental Manager shall sign off the Audit Report when all short-term actions have been carried out and all long-term actions have been notified.

The Environmental Manager shall progress long-term actions and record progress on the Corrective/Preventive Action Form. The form shall be signed off when all actions are complete.

The Environmental Manager shall in due course verify that actions have been effective, and sign off the verification box.

10. Report to management

The Environmental Manager shall prepare a brief report summarising audits carried out, the findings and resulting corrective actions and submit it to each environmental management review meeting for discussion.

(Author's note: The schedule in Annex A has spare lines under the heading Operational Procedures (ISO 14001 Clause 4.4.6). This is to allow for the fact that you will probably have more Operating Procedures associated with this clause than can be audited in one session. Therefore divide the procedures into sensible groups, and make each group an audit topic in its own right. The same situation may apply to emergencies.)

Operating Procedure 21:   Issue . . . . . .
Dated . . . . / . . . . /200 . . . .
Page: 3 of 3

ENVIRONMENTAL AUDIT TOPICS

Topic	ISO 14001 Clause	Manual ref.	Related documents
Environmental management system	4.1	1	
Environmental policy	4.2	2	
Environmental aspects	4.3.1	3.1	
Legal requirements	4.3.2	3.2	
Objectives, targets, management programme	4.3.3, 4.3.4	3.3, 3.4	
Structure and responsibility	4.4.1	4.1	
Training, awareness and competence	4.4.2	4.2	
Communication	4.4.3	4.3	
Documentation, document control	4.4.4, 4.4.5	4.4, 4.5	
Operational control	4.4.6	4.6	
Emergencies	4.4.7	4.7	
Monitoring and measurement	4.5.1	5.1	
Nonconformance, corrective & preventive action	4.5.2	5.2	
Records	4.5.3	5.3	
EMS audits	4.5.4	5.4	
Management review	4.6	6	

Annex A Oper Proc 21: Issue . . . . . .

Dated . . . . / . . . . /200 . . . .

Page: 1 of 1

SCHEDULE OF ENVIRONMENTAL AUDITS
YEAR 200. . . .

Topic	Jan	Feb	Mar	Apr	May	Jun	Jly	Aug	Sep	Oct	Nov	Dec
Environmental management system												
Environmental policy												
Environmental aspects												
Legal requirements												
Objectives, targets, management programme												
Structure and responsibility												
Training, awareness and competence												
Communication												
Documentation, document control												
Operational control												
Emergencies												
Monitoring and measurement												
Nonconformance, corrective & preventive action												
Records												
EMS audits												
Management review												

☐ Audit planned

☒ Audit taken place (no action required)

◪ Action required

▨ Short-term action taken, long-term action notified

Signed: .... Date: ....

Annex B Oper Proc 21:   Issue . . . . . .

Dated . . . . / . . . . /200. . . .

Page: 1 of 1

AUDIT FINDINGS

Scope/subject:	Contact:	Auditors:	Date:	Audit no:	Page:	of

Ref.	Evidence and findings	Recommendations for action	Status	Action taken/notified

Short-term action taken, long-term action notified: ....

Environmental Manager .... Date: ....

Annex C Oper Proc 21: Issue ....
Dated ..../..../200.....

Page: 1 of 1

CORRECTIVE/PREVENTIVE ACTION FORM

To:	Date:
Subject:	Ref:
Action Requested:	Target Completion Date:

Date:	Progress:

Action complete:	Signature: Date:
Effectiveness verified:	Signature: Date:

Circulation:

Annex D Oper Proc 21:   Issue . . . . . .

Dated . . . . / . . . . /200 . . . .

Page: 1 of 1

Operating Procedure No. 22

Management review

(Author's note: If you have an ISO 9001 quality system you will already be holding management reviews of quality performance. In this instance, I do not recommend that you bring together environmental and quality functions into one procedure. Management needs to keep a clear head about both subjects and it is possible that different people will be needed at the meetings. So keep this Operating Procedure separate from any corresponding quality procedure.)

1. Purpose and scope

This procedure sets out the requirements of management review, whereby top management ensures environmental performance and the structure of the environmental management system (EMS) including the environmental policy are kept up-to-date so that the organisation complies with the law and identifies and keeps its environmental aspects under control.

2. Responsibility

The Managing Director is responsible for chairing environmental management review meetings.

The Environmental Manager is responsible for convening meetings, preparing and distributing the agenda, preparing and circulating minutes and action plans, and following up to ensure that action plans are completed.

3. Environmental management review meetings

3.1 Frequency and purpose

Environmental management review meetings shall be held every 3 months (OR 4 months, OR 6 months OR 12 months) to review the environmental management system to ensure its continuing suitability for the needs and objectives of the organisation, and its adequacy and effectiveness, and to set and progress environmental objectives and targets.

3.2 Attendees

The meetings shall be attended by:

- The Managing Director (in the chair).
- The Environmental Manager.
- (list the other people who need to be present at every meeting, e.g. production director/manager, technical director/manager).

Other managers and staff shall attend the meeting if required by the agenda.

3.3 Agenda

The following standard agenda shall apply. Other items shall be added as appropriate.

Every meeting

- Review of any actions outstanding from previous meetings.
- Review of environmental performance arising from nonconformities and incidents, complaints and audit findings.
- Confirmation of preventive actions if necessary.
- Review of progress towards the achievement of the current programme of improvement objectives and targets.
- Review of the Environmental Policy, Environmental Management Manual and Operating Procedures to ensure that they are still consistent with, and relevant to, the overall policies and objectives of the organisation.

Annually

- Review of the Register of Environmental Aspects and their relative environmental impacts, leading to the setting of improvement objectives and targets for the coming year (see Operating Procedure 13).
- Setting of improvement action plans for the coming year.
- Review of environmental training needs.

3.4 Follow-up

The Environmental Manager shall write minutes of the meeting including the action points and names of people responsible for action. The minutes shall be distributed to all concerned.

The Environmental Manager shall follow-up the actions and sign them off on his or her copy of the minutes when they have been completed.

Operating Procedure 22: Issue . . . . . .

Dated . . . . /. . . . /200 . . . .

Page: 2 of 2

Environmental Management Manual

A.J. Edwards

Introduction

This model Environmental Management Manual has been written to show how to describe the structure and content of an environmental management system and to demonstrate that the organisation has satisfied all the requirements of ISO 14001.

The word 'organisation' has been used throughout to describe your business, firm or company. I suggest you change this to 'company', 'firm', 'practice', etc., as appropriate. This will give a greater sense of identity to the reader. Where '. . . . . . Ltd' is written, I suggest you insert the actual name of your organisation.

As in the other documents in this set, possible alternative text is shown (OR . . . . . .). Optional text is shown in brackets.

All the operative clauses of ISO 14001 are in Section 4 of the published Standard. Some people therefore choose to number the sections of their Manual 4.2, 4.5.1, etc. There is a presentational advantage in keeping the numbering as simple as possible. Therefore in this model Manual the initial 4 has been omitted, e.g. Clause 4.2 of the Standard has been numbered 2, Clause 4.5.1 has been numbered 5.1.

This text is available on the accompanying website. It can be downloaded and modified as required.

Contents

. . . . . . Ltd

ENVIRONMENTAL POLICY

The management and all who work at . . . . . . Ltd are committed to the care of the environment and the prevention of pollution.

The organisation ensures that all its activities are carried out in conformance with the relevant environmental legislation (and the Code of Practice issued by the . . . . . . Trade Association OR . . . . . .).

(The organisation operates processes which are prescribed under the Environmental Protection Act 1990: Part 1 (OR Pollution Prevention and Control Act 1999), and observes the requirements laid down by . . . . . . County Council (OR the Environment Agency).)

The organisation seeks to minimise waste arisings, promote recycling, reduce energy consumption, reduce harmful emissions and, where possible, to work with suppliers who themselves have sound environmental policies.

An essential feature of the environmental management system is a commitment to improving environmental performance. This is achieved by setting annual environmental improvement objectives and targets which are regularly monitored and reviewed. The objectives and targets are publicised throughout the organisation and all staff are committed to their achievement.

(In particular . . . . . . (you may wish to include reference to the control of the most important aspects, or to the most significant of the current list of environmental objectives).)

In order to ensure the achievement of the above commitments, the organisation has implemented an environmental management system which satisfies the requirements of BS EN ISO 14001: 1996.

This Policy and the obligations and responsibilities required by the environmental management system have been communicated to all employees. The Policy is available to the public on request.

Managing Director   Date

Environmental Management Manual
Issue . . . . . .   Revision . . . . . .
Dated . . . . /. . . . /200. . . .
Page: 1 of 16

0. Introduction to . . . . . Ltd

. . . . . . Ltd is a (describe the type of organisation, e.g. engineering company, plastic injection moulding company, transport company, firm of solicitors, etc.) specialising in (give more detail of the main type of product or service). It has been trading since . . . . . . (and is a subsidiary of . . . . . .).

The organisation is located in/at . . . . . . and currently employs approximately . . . . . . people.

The main processes are . . . . . . (Also state if any of these processes are regulated by the Environment Agency or local authority under the Environmental Protection Act 1990: Part 1 (OR Pollution Prevention and Control Act 1999).)

(If appropriate, mention principal customers).

. . . . . . Ltd is committed to protecting the environment, and to this end has created and implemented an environmental management system which is described in this Environmental Management Manual.

(The organisation is registered to the quality management Standard ISO 9001, and where possible the requirements of ISO 14001 and ISO 9001 have been integrated into a common management system.)

Environmental Management Manual

Issue . . . . . .   Revision . . . . . .

Dated . . . . /. . . . /200 . . . .

Page: 2 of 16

1. Environmental management system

As required by Clause 4.1 of the Standard, ... Ltd has created and implemented an environmental management system (EMS) which conforms to the requirements of BS EN ISO 14001: 1996, hereafter referred to as ISO 14001.

The EMS is structured by means of the following documents:

- Environmental Policy.
- Environmental Manual.
- Registers of Environmental Aspects and Environmental Legislation.
- Operating Procedures.
- (Work Instructions.)

Environmental Management Manual
Issue ...... Revision ......
Dated ..../..../200....
Page: 3 of 16

2. Environmental policy

As required by Clause 4.2 of the Standard, ... Ltd's commitment to the environment is set out in the Environmental Policy. The Policy is signed by the Managing Director, is displayed on the notice board and has been communicated to all employees. The policy statement is printed at the front of this Manual.

The Policy is supported by specific objectives and targets which are reviewed annually.

3. Planning

3.1 Environmental aspects

As required by Clause 4.3.1 of the Standard, the organisation has examined its activities and products (OR services) to determine which of them have an impact on the environment, and where possible the impact has been measured. The results of the analysis are presented in a Register of Environmental Aspects.

The relative significance of the various aspects is a factor that influences the selection of items for inclusion in environmental improvement and action plans. Guidance on how to rate the significance of aspects is given in Operating Procedure 13 'Environmental objectives and targets'.

The information on environmental aspects is reviewed and updated as part of the internal environmental audit programme (see paragraph 5.4).

3.2 Legal and other requirements

As required by Clause 4.3.2 of the Standard, the organisation has determined which environmental legislation and regulations and any relevant codes of practice apply to its activities. The information on legal and other requirements is presented in a Register of Environmental Legislation.

Operating Procedure 17 'Document control' contains instructions on how to keep the Register up-to-date.

If changes to legislation require the organisation to make changes in the way it operates, the relevant Operating Procedures will be revised or new Procedures will be written.

3.3 Objectives and targets

As required by Clause 4.3.3 of the Standard, the organisation sets environmental improvement objectives and targets. Annually, the Managing Director at an environmental management review meeting reviews the information contained in the Registers of Environmental Aspects and Environmental Legislation, and selects which items shall be adopted as objectives and targets for the coming year.

In setting these objectives and targets, the organisation is mindful of:

- The Environmental Policy.
- The relative importance of the environmental aspects.
- Relevant legislation, etc.
- The view of any interested parties.
- The need to prevent pollution in general.

Environmental Management Manual

Issue . . . . . .   Revision . . . . . .

Dated . . . . / . . . . /200 . . . .

Page: 5 of 16

Operating Procedure 13 'Environmental objectives and targets' describes the process of evaluating and ranking environmental aspects.

3.4 Environmental management programme

As required by Clause 4.3.4 of the Standard, each objective or target is set out in an environmental action plan which states the objective of the plan, who shall be responsible for managing the project, and the stages and timescale.

The progress of environmental action plans is monitored by the Environmental Manager and is reviewed at subsequent environmental management review meetings.

The process is described in Operating Procedure 13 'Environmental objectives and targets'.

When new products and processes are being developed, Operating Procedure 14 'New products and processes' requires an assessment of the environmental implications of the development.

Specific Operating Procedures are introduced when they are needed to ensure the adequate implementation of any part of the environmental programme.

Environmental Management Manual
Issue . . . . . .   Revision . . . . . .
Dated . . . . / . . . . /200 . . . .
Page: 6 of 16

4. Implementation and operation

4.1 Structure and responsibility

As required by Clause 4.4.1 of the Standard, the Managing Director (OR the organisation) has set up a management structure and has allocated responsibilities for environmental activities so that there is effective management of the EMS.

The organisation's management structure is shown in the chart on the next page. The responsibilities of individual jobs which have an input to environmental performance are described in the following paragraphs.

The Managing Director also ensures that adequate resources in terms of people, skills and equipment are available to allow the proper exercise of these responsibilities.

(Author's note: The following paragraphs describe job responsibilities as they might apply in order to implement the model EMS set out in this Manual and the accompanying Operating Procedures. The best way to approach tackling this part of the Manual is to look through your Operating Procedures; if a job title appears in the 'responsibilities' paragraph, that job needs to appear here.)

Managing Director

The Managing Director has overall responsibility for the policies and activities of the organisation. He or she chairs the environmental management review meetings, has the ultimate responsibility for setting environmental objectives and targets, and authorises the Environmental Policy.

All Directors and Managers

All Directors and Managers are committed to the Environmental Policy.

They are responsible for ensuring that they and their staff are aware of the requirements of the EMS and for training them in the specific environmental responsibilities of each job.

Environmental 'management representative'

The Managing Director has appointed a senior manager who, in addition to his or her other responsibilities, acts as the 'management representative' with responsibility for ensuring that the requirements of the Standard are implemented and maintained. This person is called the Environmental Manager.

The Environmental Manager's responsibilities are:

- To set up the EMS in accordance with the requirements of ISO 14001.
- To keep the EMS up to date.

<table>
<tr><td>Environmental Management Manual</td></tr>
<tr><td>Issue . . . . . .   Revision . . . . . .</td></tr>
<tr><td>Dated . . . . /. . . . /200 . . . .</td></tr>
<tr><td>Page: 7 of 16</td></tr>
</table>

ENVIRONMENTAL ORGANISATION CHART

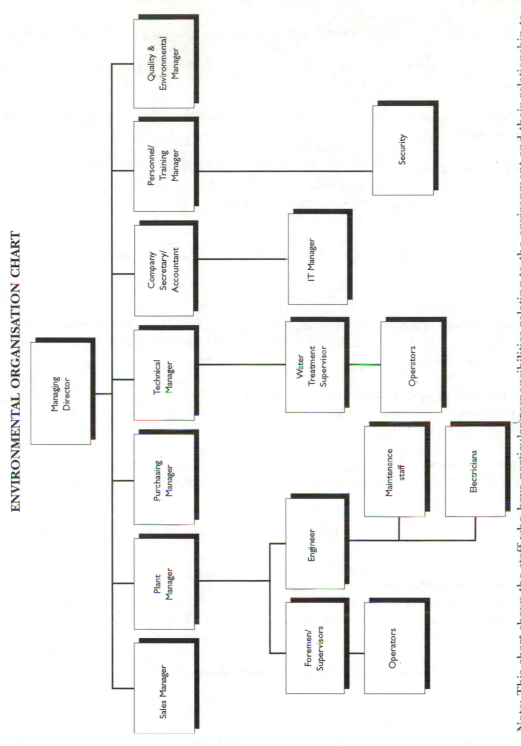

Note: This chart shows the staff who have particular responsibilities relating to the environment and their relationship to each other. It does not show relative status levels.

Environmental Management Manual

Issue ...... Revision ......

Dated ..../..../200....

Page: 8 of 16

235

- To obtain authorisation of environmental documentation and to control its distribution and revision.
- To keep environmental records.
- To monitor the progress towards the attainment of environmental objectives and targets.
- Dealings with statutory bodies.
- Environmental awareness training.
- To arrange internal environmental audits.
- To report on environmental performance to the management environmental review meeting.

Plant Manager

The Plant Manager is responsible for the control of the environmental aspects related to all manufacturing activities and for emergency procedures.

Engineer

The Engineer and staff are responsible for maintaining plant and equipment so that it performs reliably.

Foremen/Supervisors

Foremen have direct control of all operating activities and are responsible for ensuring that their staff observe the Operating Procedures. They are the first line of defence in the event of an environmental incident.

Technical Manager and Water Treatment Supervisor

The Technical Manager has overall responsibility and the Water Treatment Supervisor has day-to-day responsibility for the performance of the water treatment plant.

Company Secretary/Accountant

The Company Secretary/Accountant is responsible for the organisation's fleet of vehicles.

IT Manager

The IT Manager is responsible for the regular back-up of computer records and their secure storage.

Personnel/Training Manager

The Training Manager is responsible for ensuring that job training in environmental responsibilities is carried out and that training records are kept.

Security

Security staff carry out environmental checks on emissions.

4.2 Training, awareness and competence

As required by Clause 4.4.2 of the Standard, all staff and new recruits receive environmental awareness training which includes the Environmental Policy, the major environmental impacts of the organisation's activities and an introduction to the EMS.

Environmental Management Manual
Issue . . . . . .   Revision . . . . . .
Dated . . . . / . . . . /200 . . . .
Page: 9 of 16

All staff are trained in the specific environmental impacts and responsibilities of their jobs, in emergency procedures and in the potential consequences of departing from the specific procedures. Where a job has the potential to cause significant environmental impacts, care is taken that job holders are competent to do the job.

Training needs are identified and the training is provided. Training records are kept.

Operating Procedure 15 'Environmental training' applies.

4.3 Communication

As required by Clause 4.4.3 of the Standard, procedures have been implemented for receiving, documenting and responding to communications from external sources on environmental subjects including complaints and requests for information.

The requirements of the EMS are communicated to staff through training and the distribution of Operating Procedures (and Work Instructions). Any matter requiring immediate attention is notified to staff by memo.

The organisation has decided to make information on its significant environmental aspects publicly available (OR . . . has decided not to make . . . . . but will respond to requests for information).

Operating Procedure 16 'Environmental communications' applies.

4.4 Environmental management system documentation

As described in Section 1 of the Manual and as required by Clause 4.4.4 of the Standard, ... Ltd has established a two (OR three) level EMS, namely:

- The Manual.
- Operating Procedures.
- (Work Instructions.)

supported by:

- The Register of Environmental Aspects.
- The Register of Environmental Legislation.

Appendix A contains a cross-referencing of the clauses of the Standard to the paragraphs of this Manual, the Operating Procedures and other relevant documents.

(Some parts of the environmental programme are administered in a similar way to the corresponding part of the organisation's quality management system. In these cases Operating Procedures have been written which apply to both environment and quality.)

4.5 Document control

As required by Clause 4.4.5 of the Standard, Operating Procedures have been implemented for controlling all the documents which comprise the documented EMS, so that:

- They can be located.
- They are reviewed and revised as necessary.

Environmental Management Manual
Issue . . . . . .   Revision . . . . . .
Dated . . . . /. . . . /200 . . . .
Page: 10 of 16

- They are authorised before release and are circulated to named people or locations.
- Obsolete documents are removed from the locations where they are used.
- Documents which need to be retained for historical or legal purposes are clearly marked as withdrawn.
- (Where documents are held on computer for direct reference, any printed copy is automatically classified as 'uncontrolled'.)

Operating Procedure 17 'Document control' refers.

Documents to be retained and their retention times are listed in Operating Procedure 20 'Environmental records'.

4.6 Operational control

As required by Clause 4.4.6 of the Standard, Operating Procedures have been written and implemented where they are needed to ensure compliance with the Environmental Policy, legal requirements, control of significant environmental aspects and progressing the environmental improvement plan.

The following Operating Procedures relate to the control of operations:

Operating Procedure
1   Disposal of controlled waste
2   Disposal of special wastes
3   Waste handling and segregation
4   Control of solvents and emissions
5   Furnace operations
6   Water treatment plant
7   Packaging
8   Storage, housekeeping and drainage
9   Maintenance
10   Environmental aspects of suppliers and subcontractors
11   Energy control and monitoring
12   Company cars

4.7 Emergency preparedness and response

As required by Clause 4.4.7 of the Standard, possible emergency situations have been identified and Operating Procedures written to keep control of the situation and to overcome any consequential environmental impacts. Some of these procedures already exist as separate documents and are referenced here. In other cases, emergency conditions are identified within Operating Procedures.

Operating Procedure
6   Water treatment plant
8   Storage, housekeeping and drainage
–   Action in case of fire
–   COMAH emergency plan

Where necessary, the procedures contain a requirement for emergency action to be tested.

Environmental Management Manual
Issue . . . . . .   Revision . . . . . .
Dated . . . . / . . . . /200 . . . .
Page: 11 of 16

5. Checking and corrective action

5.1 Monitoring and measurement

As required by Clause 4.5.1 of the Standard, monitoring and measurement activities are controlled as follows:

- Internal auditors are required to draw attention to any environmental aspect which they feel is not adequately represented or controlled in the EMS. Operating Procedure 21 'Internal environmental audits' refers.
- The action plans leading to the achievement of environmental objectives and targets are regularly reviewed to ensure that satisfactory progress is being made. Operating Procedure 13 'Environmental objectives and targets' refers.
- Monitoring and measuring equipment which is used to control or measure environmental operations or performance is regularly calibrated and records are kept. Operating Procedure 18 'Monitoring and measuring equipment' refers.
- How the organisation complies with relevant legislation has been incorporated into Operating Procedures. Compliance is therefore tested as part of the internal auditing of these procedures. Operating Procedure 21 refers.

5.2 Nonconformance, corrective and preventive action

As required by Clause 4.5.2 of the Standard, any nonconformance or incident with environmental significance is recorded and investigated, steps are taken to control any impact caused, and when appropriate and depending on the seriousness of the incident, corrective or preventive action is taken to prevent a recurrence. When necessary, Operating Procedures will be revised or new procedures written.

Environmental incidents may arise from:

- A failure to observe Operating Procedures.
- Inadequate Operating Procedures.
- Unforeseen circumstances e.g. abnormal operating conditions.
- Emergencies.
- Complaints.

Operating Procedure 19 'Nonconformance, corrective and preventive action' refers.

5.3 Records

As required by Clause 4.5.3 of the Standard, all documents and records which form part of the EMS are defined, identified, collated, indexed, filed and stored securely so that they will not deteriorate and can be retrieved. Retention times are defined.

Back-up procedures are implemented for records held on computer.

Operating Procedure 20 'Environmental records' refers.

5.4 Environmental management system audit

As required by Clause 4.5.4 of the Standard, internal environmental audits are carried out to determine that the EMS has been properly implemented and maintained and that it conforms to the requirements of the Standard.

Auditors are appointed and trained. An audit schedule is prepared annually so that every audit topic is audited at least once a year; the frequency of audits depends on the importance of the topic and the outcome of previous audits. Audits are planned to examine each aspect of the relevant part of the Manual and the related Operating Procedures (and Work Instructions).

Auditors are also required to be alert to the environmental impact of the activities they are auditing and to draw attention to any aspect which they feel is not adequately represented or controlled in the EMS.

Audit reports are written and recommendations for corrective or preventive action are made and agreed when necessary which are implemented and followed up.

Audit findings and actions taken are reported to the environmental management review meetings.

Operating Procedure 21 'Internal environmental audits' refers.

Environmental Management Manual
Issue . . . . . .   Revision . . . . . .
Dated . . . . /. . . . /200 . . . .
Page: 13 of 16

6. Management review

As required by Clause 4.6 of the Standard, the Managing Director and other Directors/ (Senior) Managers meet every 3 months (OR 4 months OR 6 months OR 12 months) to review the EMS to ensure its continuing suitability for the needs and objectives of the organisation, and its adequacy and effectiveness. The meeting also sets and progresses environmental objectives and targets.

The agenda includes the following items:

- Review of any actions outstanding from previous meetings.
- Review of environmental performance arising from nonconformities and incidents, complaints and audit findings.
- Confirmation of preventive actions.
- Review of progress towards the achievement of environmental objectives and targets.
- Review of the Environmental Policy, Environmental Management Manual and Operating Procedures to ensure they are still consistent with, and relevant to, the overall policies and objectives of the organisation.
- Review of the Register of Environmental Aspects and their relative environmental impacts, leading to the setting of new environmental objectives and targets.
- Setting improvement action plans.
- Review of environmental training needs.

Notes of action points are distributed and followed-up to completion.
Operating Procedure 22 'Management review' refers.

Appendix A

STRUCTURE OF THE ENVIRONMENTAL MANAGEMENT SYSTEM

Clause of ISO 14001	Title	Manual paragraph no	Related documents
4.1	**Environmental management system**	1	–
4.2	**Environmental policy**	2	–
4.3	**Planning**		
4.3.1	Environmental aspects	3.1	Register of Environmental Aspects OP 13 Environmental objectives and targets
4.3.2	Legal and other requirements	3.2	Register of Environmental Legislation OP 17 Document control
4.3.3	Objectives and targets	3.3	OP 13 Environmental objectives and targets
4.3.4	Environmental management program	3.4	OP 13 Environmental objectives and targets
4.4	**Implementation and operation**		
4.4.1	Structure and responsibility	4.1	–
4.4.2	Training, awareness and competence	4.2	OP 15 Environmental training
4.4.3	Communication	4.3	OP 16 Environmental Communications
4.4.4	EMS documentation	4.4	–
4.4.5	Document control	4.5	OP 17 Document control

242

4.4.6	Operational control	4.6	OP 1 Disposal of controlled waste OP 2 Disposal of special waste OP 3 Waste handling and segregation OP 4 Control of solvents and emissions OP 5 Furnace operations OP 6 Water treatment plant OP 7 Packaging OP 8 Storage, housekeeping and drainage OP 9 Maintenance OP 10 Environmental aspects of suppliers and subcontractors OP 11 Energy control and monitoring OP 12 Company cars
4.4.7	Emergency procedures and response	4.7	OP 6 Water treatment plant OP 8 Storage, housekeeping and drainage Action in case of fire COMAH emergency plan
4.5	**Checking and corrective action**		
4.5.1	Monitoring and measurement	5.1	OP 13 Environmental objectives and targets OP 18 Monitoring and measuring equipment OP 21 Internal environmental audits
4.5.2	Non-conformance and corrective and preventive action	5.2	OP 19 Nonconformance, corrective and preventive action
4.5.3	Records	5.3	OP 20 Environmental records
4.5.4	EMS audit	5.4	OP 21 Internal environmental audits
4.6	**Management review**	6	OP 22 Management review

Index

Index